FRENCH WOMEN DON'T GET FAT

French Women

Don't Get Fat

MIREILLE GUILIANO

ALFRED A. KNOPF   NEW YORK   2005

THIS IS A BORZOI BOOK PUBLISHED BY ALFRED A. KNOPF

Library of Congress Cataloging-in-Publication Data
Guiliano, Mireille, [date].
French women don't get fat / Mireille Guiliano
p.   cm.
ISBN 1-4000-4212-7
1. Reducing diets.   2. Women—Health and hygiene—France.
3. Food habits—France.   4. Food—Psychological aspects.   I. Title.
RM222.2.G785 2004
613.2'5—dc22   2004048424

Printed in the United States of America
Published January 4, 2005
Reprinted Three Times
Fifth Printing, January 2005

*Proceeds from this book are being donated to
charities in education and the arts.*

What is more important than the meal? Doesn't the least observant [wo]man-about-town look upon the implementation and ritual progress of a meal as a liturgical prescription? Isn't all of civilization apparent in these careful preparations, which consecrate the spirit's triumph over a raging appetite?

—*Valéry*

CONTENTS

FRENCH WOMEN DON'T GET FAT

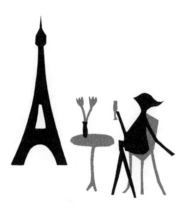

Whatever the state of Franco-American relations—admittedly a bit frayed from time to time—we should not lose sight of the singular achievements of French civilization. Until now, I humbly submit, one glorious triumph has remained largely unacknowledged, yet it's a basic and familiar anthropological truth: French women don't get fat.

I am no physician, physiologist, psychologist, nutritionist, or any manner of "-ist" who helps or studies people professionally. I was, however, born and raised in France, and with two good eyes I've been observing the French for a lifetime. Plus, I eat a lot. One can find exceptions, as with any rule, but overwhelmingly, French women do as I do: they eat as they like and don't get fat. *Pourquoi?*

Over the past decade, we Americans have made valuable progress in understanding the French capacity for getting away with murder vis-à-vis food and drink. The cautious acknowledgment of a "French Paradox," for example, has sent countless heart patients and wellness enthusiasts sprinting to the wine store for bottles of red. But otherwise, the wisdom of the French way of eating and living, and in particular the uncanny power of French women to stay svelte, remains little understood, much less exploited. With myself as living proof, I have successfully counseled dozens of American women over the years, including some who have come to work for me at Clicquot, Inc., in New York City. I've also addressed thousands on aspects of this subject in talks. I've been teased by American friends and business associates: "When will you write zee book?" Well, *le jour est arrivé!*

Could it be Nature alone? Could the slow wheel of evolution have had time enough to create a discrete gene pool of slender women? *J'en doute.* No, French women have a *system,* their *trucs*—a collection of well-honed tricks. Though I was born into it, living happily as a child and even a teenager by what my *maman* taught me, at a moment in my adolescence the wheels came off. In America as an exchange student, I suffered a catastrophe that I was totally unprepared for: a twenty-pound catastrophe. It sent me into a wilderness from which I had to find my way back. Fortunately, I had help: a family physician whom I still call Dr. Miracle. He led me to rediscover my hereditary French gastronomic wisdom and to recover my former shape. (Yes, this is an American story, too, a parable of fall and redemption.)

I have now lived and worked in America most of my life.

(I like to believe that I embody the best parts of being American and being French.) I moved here a few years after university and worked as a UN translator, then for the French government, promoting French food and wine. I married a wonderful American and eventually found my way to corporate life. In 1984, I took the leap that has let me live in two cultures ever since. The venerable Champagne House of Veuve Clicquot, founded in 1772, boldly opened a U.S. subsidiary to handle the importation and marketing of Champagne Veuve Clicquot and other fine wines. As the first employee, I immediately became the highest-ranking woman on staff since Madame Clicquot, who died in 1866. Today I am a CEO and director of Champagne Veuve Clicquot, part of the luxury-goods group LVMH.

All the while, I've continued to practice what most French women do without a second thought. And the dangers I have faced for years now are well above average. No exaggeration, my business requires me to eat in restaurants about three hundred times a year (tough job, I know, but someone has to do it). I've been at it for twenty years, never without a glass of wine or Champagne at my side (business is business). These are full meals: no single course of frisée salad and sparkling water for me. Yet I repeat: I am not overweight or unhealthy. This book aims to explain how I do it and, more important, how you can, too. By learning and practicing the way French women traditionally think and act in relation to food and life, you too can do what might seem impossible. What's the secret? First, a word about what it's not.

So many of us do double duty, working harder inside and outside the home than most men will ever know. On top of it, we must find a way to stay healthy as we try to maintain an appearance that pleases us. But let's face it: more than half of us cannot maintain a stable, healthy weight even with all the self-inflicted deprivation we can muster. Sixty-five percent of Americans are overweight, and the fastest-selling books are diet books, most of them now written like biochemistry manuals. No matter how many appear, there are always ten more on the way. Could dietary technology really be progressing as fast as the marketing? Anyway, the demand persists. Why? Why don't the million-copy wonders put a definitive end to our woes? Simply put, unsustainable extremism.

Most diet books are based on radical programs. Apart from a brief Jacobin interlude in the eighteenth century, extremism has never been the French way. America, however, gravitates toward different philosophies, quick fixes, and extreme measures. In diet as in other matters, these work for a time, but they're no way to live. You're bound to slip out of your Zone, fall off your Pyramid, lose count of your calories. And why not? *C'est normal!* It doesn't help matters that one extreme prescription is often contradicted by the very next one to gain traction. Who doesn't remember the high-carb days? Or the grapefruit days? Now everything's fat and protein, and carbs are the devil; first dairy products are your worst enemy, then they are the only thing you can eat. Ditto wine, bran, red meat. The unstated principle seems to be, if you bore yourself to death with one kind of food group, eventually you'll lose interest in eating altogether and the pounds will come off. In some cases, they do. But what happens after you stop the radical program? You know what happens. For this reason, *attention!* Banish the diet book! You don't need an ideology or a technology, you need what French women have: a balanced and time-tested relation to food and life. Finally, the coup de grâce against these extreme programs is their general lack of attention to the individuality of our metabolisms. Written mostly by men, they rarely acknowledge that the physiology of women is profoundly different. And a woman's metabolism changes over time: a woman of twenty-five with some weight to lose faces a different challenge from that of a fifty-year-old.

While my stories and lessons can be of benefit to anyone, this book is intended primarily for women, being based solely on my experience as a woman. It's not only for Americans, but for women throughout the developed world, who face career pressures, personal stress, globalization, and all the traps of twenty-first-century society. And it is not for those whose weight is an immediate health risk, or who require a medically prescribed diet. I speak specifically to women who need to lose up to thirty pounds, which is a great proportion of the population. Nevertheless, like the *Tintin* cartoons, the story is for all ages, seven to seventy-seven, and I offer advice for tailoring it to the various periods of our lives. Since French women do not live by bread alone, much less high protein, I present a comprehensive approach to living, strategies and philosophy you can make your own, including menus and quick recipes anyone can follow and, *bien sûr,* a guide to how we move. Oh, and I like to think that men of all nations could benefit from learning a thing or two about the other gender.

Okay, so what are the secrets of French women? How do we account for all those middle-aged women with the figures of twenty-five-year-olds strolling the boulevards of Paris? The following chapters draw on observations from my time in Paris (about twelve weeks a year) compared with my weeks in New York City and around the United States and the world. I invite the reader to reflect on the differences and modify her approach to healthy living accordingly.

At the outset, let's state that French women simply do not suffer the terror of kilos that afflicts so many of their American sisters. All the chatter about diets I hear at cocktail parties in America would make any French woman cringe. In France, we don't talk about "diets," certainly not with strangers. We may eventually share a trick or two we've learned with a very close friend—some cunning refinement of an old French principle. But mainly we spend our social time talking about what we enjoy: feelings, family, hobbies, philosophy, politics, culture, and, yes, food, especially food (but never diets).

French women take pleasure in staying thin by eating well, while Americans typically see it as a conflict and obsess over it. French women don't skip meals or substitute slimming shakes for them. They have two or three courses at lunch and then another three (sometimes four) at dinner. And with wine, *bien sûr*. How do they do it? Well, that's a story. That's the story. One hint: They eat with their heads, and they do not leave the table feeling stuffed or guilty.

Learning that less *can* be more and discovering *how* one can eat everything in moderation are keys. So are exertion in proportion to calories consumed and a much more plentiful intake of water. We no longer work eighteen hours a day in a mine or on a farm, and our Paleolithic hunter-gatherer days are long past. Nevertheless, most Americans eat at least 10 to 30 percent more than needed, not to survive but to satisfy psychological hunger. The trick is to manage and gratify your appetites, while determining how, when, and what to reduce. The wonderful feelings of satisfaction you'll notice when a new menu is introduced—a heightened enjoyment even as overall intake is decreased—will then inspire you to continue along the wellness road. It's all a matter of learning the most basic of French rules: Fool yourself.

Many nutritionists (valuable educators) promote a commonsense approach but charge a fortune to tell you how to implement it. The money spent on attempting to lose weight is out of all proportion with outcomes. Most women simply can't afford to see a doctor or nutritionist, join a health club, go to a spa, or have meals delivered. What will it cost you to practice the secrets of French women? Well, above the cost of this book, very little. My do-it-yourself approach is within virtually every woman's means. The only equipment is a small scale to weigh some of your foods during the critically important first three months. You might also want to buy a yogurt machine if you want to eat *le vrai yaourt,* a key element in my lifestyle program; and if you are past age forty, you should acquire some dumbbells for strength building. *C'est tout.*

I begin with my childhood in France and then share my experience as a young woman with a weight challenge. Faced with the first physical wake-up call of my life, I turned to traditional French principles for help. By sharing my experience not only with food, but with a "total approach" to healthy living, I aim to guide each reader toward finding her own *equilibrium.* (*Le mot juste* indeed: it's an important concept, because while our bodies are machines, no two are built exactly alike, and they "reset" themselves repeatedly over time. A program that doesn't evolve with you will not see you through the long run.) I provide menus you can follow exactly, but the goal is to develop what works for you as you cultivate a new intuition. I'm not presenting prescriptions so much as templates. Tailor them according to your preferences, paying attention to your own body, schedule, environment, and other unique characteristics. In fact, my emphasis is on the simplicity, flexibility, and *rewards* of doing it yourself. This fine-tuning can't be done by a doctor-author who's never met you.

As I recount my own story from adolescent meltdown to rescue to a new approach that has worked for decades and counting, I lay out a path for you. I take readers through a complete program:

Phase one, *wake-up call:* an old-fashioned three-week inventory of meals. A clear-eyed look at what you're eating, which itself, even after a couple of days, can begin your turnaround.

Phase two, *recasting:* an introduction to the French school of portions and diversity of nourishment. You'll identify and temporarily suspend some key food "offenders." This is usually a three-month process, though for some a month will do the trick. It won't be a dietary boot camp, merely a chance for your body to recalibrate. There is discipline, but flexibility is vitally important, especially at this key motivational stage: the value of avoiding routine both in meals and in activities, emphasizing quality over quantity. No pizza three days in a row, but also no three hours at the gym on Saturday. You'll acclimate with your five senses to a new gastronomy (a Greek word, even before it was a French one, meaning "rules of the stomach"). Three months is not a short time, but neither is it long for something you'll never need to do again. Naturally, it takes longer to reset your body's dials than to lose seven pounds of water, the initial part of many extremist diets. But because it is French, there will be pleasures, lots of them.

Phase three, *stabilization:* a stage wherein everything you like to eat is reintegrated in proper measure. You have already achieved your reset "equilibrium" and should be at least halfway toward your weight-loss goal. Amazingly, at this point you can increase your indulgences and continue to slim down or just maintain your equilibrium if you are already there. I give advice for practicing ideas about seasonality and seasoning, powerful tools and not nearly as much trouble as some imagine. I present more recipes based on the French knack for variations on a theme, or how to make three easy dishes out of one with delicious results, saving time, money, and calories.

Phase four, *the rest of your life:* You are at your target weight, a stable equilibrium, and the rest is just refinements. You know enough about your body and preferences to make little adjustments in the event of any unexpected drifts, especially as you enter new phases of life. Your eating and living habits are by now tailored to your tastes and metabolism, so like a classic Chanel suit, they should last you forever with minor alterations over the years. Now you will be eating in a totally different light, with an intuition to rival that of any French woman—a cultivated respect for freshness and flavor that unlocks the world of sensory delights to be discovered in presentation, color, and variety. What you do you will do for pleasure, not punishment. You'll enjoy chocolate and a glass of wine with dinner. *Pourquoi pas?*

In addition to nourishment, which is the main subject, I'll

describe aspects of healthy living that need to be pleasurable as well. As with food, these do not require extreme measures (physical, emotional, intellectual, spiritual, or financial)— only a sense of balance. They include elements of what I like to call French Zen, which can be learned quickly and easily and practiced anywhere (mainly, French women do not go to gyms, but if that is your pleasure, *à chacun son goût!*). Even the French know there is much more to life than eating, so here too you'll find the French take on other diversions, like love and laughter. From beginning to end, it will be important to recognize that Montaigne's *aperçu* is more relevant today than ever: A healthy body and healthy mind work together. To maintain both, there is no substitute for *joie de vivre* (an expression for which there is tellingly no American equivalent).

Now I have a few stories to tell, a few dozen, actually. I take pleasure in being a raconteur as well as in eating and drinking. They will drive home basic concepts, but I hope you will also enjoy them *comme ça*. Unlike a diet book, this book doesn't let you flip to graphics and jump right in: you'll have to read it. Learning to eat right is like learning a language— nothing works like immersion.

Let the tale begin.

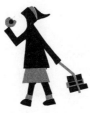

VIVE L'AMÉRIQUE:
THE BEGINNING . . . I AM OVERWEIGHT

I love my adopted homeland. But first, as an exchange student in Massachusetts, I learned to love chocolate-chip cookies and brownies. And I gained twenty pounds.

My love affair with America had begun with my love of the English language; we met at the *lycée* (junior high and high school) when I turned eleven. English was my favorite class after French literature, and I simply adored my English teacher. He had never been abroad but spoke English without a French accent or even a British one. He had learned it during World War II, when he found himself in a POW camp with a high school teacher from Weston, Massachusetts (I suspect they had long hours to practice). Without knowing whether they'd make it out alive, they decided that if they did, they would start an exchange program for high school seniors. Each year, one student from the United States would come to our town and one of us would go to Weston. The exchange continues to this day, and the competition is keen.

During my last year at the *lycée,* I had good enough grades to apply, but I wasn't interested. With dreams of becoming an English teacher or professor, I was eager to start undergraduate studies at the local university. And at eighteen, naturally I had also convinced myself I was madly in love with a boy in my town. He was the handsomest though admittedly not the brightest boy around, the *coqueluche* (the darling) of all the girls. I couldn't dream of parting from him, so I didn't even think of applying for Weston. But in the schoolyard, between classes, there was hardly another topic of conversation. Among my friends, the odds-on favorite to go was Monique; she wanted it so badly, and besides, she was the best in our class, a fact not lost on the selection committee, which was chaired by my English teacher and included among its distinguished ranks PTA members, other teachers, the mayor, and the local Catholic priest, balanced by the Protestant minister. But on the Monday morning when the announcement was expected, the only thing announced was that no decision had been made.

At home that Thursday morning (those days, there was no school on Thursdays but half days on Saturday), my English teacher appeared at the door. He had come to see my mother, which seemed rather strange, considering my good grades. As soon as he left, with a big, satisfied smile but not a word to me except hello, my mother called me. Something was *très important.*

The selection committee had not found a suitable candidate. When I asked about Monique, my mother tried to explain something not easily fathomed at my age: My friend had everything going for her, but her parents were Communists, and that would not fly in America. The committee had debated at great length (it was a small town, where everybody was fully informed about everybody else), but they could not escape concluding that a daughter of Communists could never represent France!

My teacher had proposed me as an alternative, and the other members had agreed. But since I had not even applied, he had to come and persuade my parents to let me go. My overadoring father, who would never have condoned my running away for a year, was not home. Perhaps my teacher was counting on this fact; but in any event, he managed to sell the idea to my mother. The real work then fell to her, because she had to persuade not only my father, but me as well. Not that she was without her own misgivings about seeing me go, but *Mamie* was always wise and farsighted; and she usually got her way. I was terribly anxious about what Monique would say, but once word got out, she was first to declare what a fine ambassador I would make. Apparently, Communist families were quite open and practical about such matters, and she had already been given to understand that family ideology had made her a dark horse from the start.

And so I went. It was a wonderful year—one of the best of my adolescence—and it certainly changed the course of my entire life. To a young French girl, Weston, a wealthy Boston suburb, seemed an American dream—green, manicured, spread out, with huge gorgeous homes and well-to-do, well-schooled families. There was tennis, horseback riding, swimming pools, golf, and two or three cars per family—a far, far cry from any town in eastern France, then or now. The time was so full of new, unimagined things, but finally too rich, and I don't mean demographically. For all the priceless new friends and experiences I was embracing, something else altogether, something sinister, was slowly taking shape. Almost before I could notice, it had turned into fifteen pounds, more or less . . . and quite probably more. It was August, my last month before the return voyage to France. I was in Nantucket with one of my adoptive families when I suffered the first blow: I caught a reflection of myself in a bathing suit. My American mother, who had perhaps been through something like this before with another daughter, instinctively registered my distress. A good seamstress, she bought a bolt of the most lovely linen and made me a summer shift. It seemed to solve the problem but really only bought me a little time.

In my final American weeks, I had become very sad at the thought of leaving all my new pals and relations, but I was also quite apprehensive of what my French friends and family would say at the sight of the new me. I had never mentioned the weight gain in letters and somehow managed to send photos showing me only from the waist up.

The moment of truth was approaching.

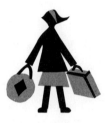

2

LA FILLE PRODIGUE:
RETURN OF THE PRODIGAL DAUGHTER

My father brought my brother with him to Le Havre to collect me. I was traveling on the SS *Rotterdam*. The ocean liner was still the transatlantic standard preferred by many French people in the late 1960s. With me was the new American exchange student from Weston, who would be spending the year in our town.

Since he had not seen me for a whole year, I expected my father, who always wore his heart on his face, would embarrass me, bounding up the gangway for the first hug and kiss. But when I spied the diminutive French man in his familiar beret—yes, a beret—he looked stunned. As I approached, now a little hesitantly, he just stared at me, and as we came near, after a few seconds that seemed endless, there in front of my brother and my American shipmate, all he could manage to say to his cherished little girl come home was, *"Tu ressembles à un sac de patates"* ("You look like a sack of potatoes"). Some things don't sound any prettier in French. I knew what he had in mind: not a market-size sack, but one of the big, 150-pound burlap affairs that are delivered to grocery stores and restaurants! Fortunately the girl from Weston spoke little French, else she would have had a troubling first impression of French family life.

At age nineteen, I could not have imagined anything more hurtful, and to this day the sting has not been topped. But my father was not being mean. True, tact was never his strength; and the teenage girl's hypersensitivity about weight and looks wasn't yet the proverbial pothole every parent today knows to steer around. The devastating welcome sprang more than anything from his having been caught off guard. Still, it was more than I could take. I was at once sad, furious, vexed, and helpless. At the time, I could not even measure the impact.

On our way home to eastern France, we stopped in Paris for a few days, just to show my friend from Weston the City of Light, but my inexorable grumpiness made everyone eager to hit the road again. I ruined Paris for all of us. I was a mess.

The coming months were bitter and awkward. I didn't want anyone to see me, but everyone wanted to greet *l'Américaine.* My mother understood right away not only how and why I had gained the weight, but also how I felt. She treaded lightly, avoiding the unavoidable topic, perhaps particularly because I had soon given her something more dire to worry about.

Having seen a bit of the world, I had lost my taste for attending the local university. I now wanted to study languages in a *Grande École* (like an Ivy League school) in Paris and, on top of that, to take a literary track at the Sorbonne at the same time. It was unusual and really an insane workload. My parents were not at all keen on the idea of Paris: if I got in (hardly a given, as the competition is legendary), it was going to be a big emotional and financial sacrifice to have me three and a half hours from home. So I had to campaign hard, but thanks in part to the obvious persistence of my raw nerves, in the end they let me go back to Paris for the famously grueling entrance exam. I passed, and in late September I moved to Paris. My parents always wanted the best for me.

By All Saints' Day (November 1), I had gained another five pounds, and by Christmas, five more still. At five feet three, I was now overweight by any standard, and nothing I owned fit, not even my American mother's summer shift. I had two flannel ones—same design, but roomier—made to cover up my lumpiness. I told the dressmaker to hurry and hated myself every minute of the day. More and more, my father's faux pas at Le Havre seemed justified. Those were blurry days of crying myself to sleep and zipping past all mirrors. It may not seem so strange an experience for a nineteen-year-old, but none of my French girlfriends was going through it.

Then something of a Yuletide miracle occurred. Or perhaps I should say, Dr. Miracle, who showed up thanks to my *mamie.* Over the long holiday break, she asked the family physician, Dr. Meyer, to pay a call. She did this most discreetly, careful not to bruise me further. Dr. Meyer had watched me grow up, and he was the kindest gentleman on earth. He assured me that getting back in shape would be really easy and just a matter of a few "old French tricks." By Easter, he promised, I'd be almost back to my old self, and certainly by the end of the school year in June I'd be ready to wear my old bathing suit, the one I'd packed for America. As in a fairy tale, it was going to be our secret. (No use boring anyone else with the particulars of our plan, he said.) And the weight would go away much faster than it came. Sounded great to me. Of course, I wanted to put my faith in Dr. Meyer, and fortunately, there didn't seem to be many options at the time.

DR. MIRACLE'S PRESCRIPTION

For the next three weeks, I was to keep a diary of *everything* I ate. This is a strategy that will sound familiar from some American diet programs, such as Weight Watchers. I was to record not only what and how much, but also when and where. There was no calorie counting, not that I could have done that. The stated purpose was simply for him to gauge the *nutritional* value of what I was eating (it was the first time I ever heard the word). Since nothing more was asked of me, I was only too happy to comply. This is the first thing you should do, too.

Dr. Meyer demanded no great precision in measurement. Just estimate, he said, stipulating "a portion" as the only unit of quantity and roughly equal to a medium-size apple. In America, where the greatest enemy of balanced eating is ever-bigger portions, I suggest a little more precision. Here's where the small kitchen scale comes in. (Bread, which sometimes comes in huge slices here, might be more easily weighed than compared with an apple, which seems bigger here, too!)

Three weeks later, I was home again for the weekend. Just before noon, Dr. Miracle, distingué, gray templed, made his second house call. He also stayed for lunch. Afterward, reviewing my diary, he immediately identified a pattern utterly obvious to him but hiding somehow from me, as I blithely recorded every crumb I put in my mouth. On the walk between school and the room I was renting in the Seventh Arrondissement, there were no fewer than sixteen pastry shops. Without my having much noticed, my meals were more and more revolving around pastry. As I was living in Paris, my family could not know this, so when I came home, my mother naturally prepared my favorites, unaware I was eating extra desserts on the sly, even under her roof.

My Parisian pastry gluttony was wonderfully diverse. In the morning there was croissant or *pain au chocolat* or *chouquette* or *tarte au sucre.* Lunch was preceded by a stop at Poîlane, the famous breadmaker's shop, where I could not resist the *pain aux raisins* or *tarte aux pommes* (apple tart) or *petits sablés.* Next stop was at a café for the ubiquitous *jambon-beurre* (ham on a buttered baguette) and what remained of the Poîlane pastry with coffee. Dinner always included and sometimes simply was an éclair, *Paris Brest, religieuse,* or *mille-feuille* (curiously called a napoleon outside France), always some form of creamy, buttery sweetness. Sometimes I would even stop off for a *palmier* (a big puff pastry sugar-covered cookie) for my *goûter* (afternoon snack). As a student, I was living off things I could eat on the go. Hardly any greens were passing my lips, and my daily serving of fruit was coming from fruit tarts. I was eating this strangely lopsided fare without the slightest thought and with utter contentment—except, of course, for how I looked.

Now this was obviously not a diet I had picked up in America, where one could hardly say the streets are lined with irresistible patisseries (though then, as now, there was no shortage of tempting hot chocolate-chip cookie stands and sellers of rich ice cream, to say nothing of a mind-boggling variety of supermarket sweets made with things infinitely worse for you than cream and butter). But as I was to learn, it was my adoptive American *way* of eating that had gone to my head and opened me up to the dangers of this delicious Parisian minefield. For in America, I had gotten into some habits: eating standing up, not making my own food, living off whatever (*n'importe quoi,* as the French say), as other kids were doing. Brownies and bagels were particular hazards; we had nothing quite like them at home, so who could tell how rich they were?

Back in France, I continued to eat *n'importe quoi,* though there were no brownies to be found. Perhaps I missed my adoptive second home and was searching for my madeleine—remembrance of sweets past. In any case, I became very free and easy with all the goodies France had to offer. Finally, I was a *mille-feuille* junkie. Like an addict's, my body came to expect too much of what had once been blissfully intoxicating in small doses.

It was time to enter rehab, but fortunately Dr. Miracle had never heard of cold turkey. (The French don't much care for *dinde* at any temperature.)

Dr. Miracle's approach was much less confrontational and more civilized. According to him, there are two selves in each of us: the one who wants to be slim and healthy and the one who wants something else. One sees the big picture—well-being, self-esteem, fitting into the latest fashions. The other wants pleasures aplenty, and now. One is Narcissus leaning over his pool; the other is Pantagruel leaning over his table. The key, he said, was not to conquer the second, but to broker a rapprochement: make friends of your two selves and be the master of both your willpower *and* your pleasures. That was the French way.

One must not forget, he said, *"il y a poids et poids"* ("there is weight and then there is weight"): there's the "ideal" body weight that shows up on insurance company charts, based on nothing but height; there is "fashion weight," an ideal much less natural, in which commerce plays a big, sometimes insidious part; and then there's the "well-being" weight, the one at which a particular individual feels *bien dans sa peau* (comfortable in his or her skin), as Montaigne says. This last concept—*bien dans sa peau*—is the one Dr. Miracle presented as our goal. It is the weight at which you can say, "I feel good and I look good." The actual number will vary at different times in our life, but invariably it is based on learning how to be a bit narcissistic while also a bit hedonistic—two notions that are not as bad or even as contradictory as many Americans suppose. (Have no fear—I do understand the Calvinist streak; my family are Huguenots—French Protestants.)

Tout est question d'équilibre (Everything is a matter of balance): this was Dr. Miracle's quintessentially French mantra. In those days it became mine as well, and so it has remained. Teaching me to find and maintain my personal equilibrium, to live *bien dans ma peau,* that was our mission.

There was nothing wrong, he explained, with eating pastries, but my consumption had gone out of balance. So for the next three months I was to pare back, finding less rich alternatives, reserving the real thing for a special treat—as it is intended. This was less deprivation than contemplation and reprogramming, because, as I would discover, achieving a balance has more to do with the mind than with the stomach; it's about discovering and dealing with *nos petits démons,* as the good doctor called them. (Once you realize that changing one's habits, like being a French woman, is mostly a state of mind, you will see why the only truly effective approach is the one that engages your head.) Later, I would be bringing back all my favorites—but in balance, enjoying them without guilt or weight gain. Easier said than done? *Peut-être.* But as we proceed, you be the judge.

Dr. Miracle was a good armchair psychologist. He recognized one valuable feature of most diets, even those that fail long-term: quick positive reinforcement. Overcoming inertia is the hardest part of changing your habits, and everyone needs a bit of early encouragement. Equilibrium must be cultivated gradually; you can't simply impose it on yourself. So I was to do something special that Saturday, to gain a head of steam for the week ahead. But thereafter I would take it one week at a time. Weekends and holidays would normally be times when I would indulge. *Gradually* even my indulgences would become savvier. Meanwhile, I would learn to balance them out through a little compensation the following week.

Dr. Miracle was something of a gourmand as well. He gave me a number of recipes, but none more important than the one for the first, and only, "tough" weekend. On reflection, it wasn't so tough at all, because of his Magical Leek Soup, a trick used by many of the local women for generations. He had prescribed it to both my mother and my grandmother at one point or another. Leeks are a mild diuretic and low in calories but highly nutritional. Forty-eight hours of leek soup plus all the water you want would provide immediate results to jump-start the recasting. For me, it was the start of a lifelong commitment to wellness as well as the beginning of my appreciation, my love, of leeks, about which there is more to say. It is a trick I still use from time to time; do try it the first weekend following your own food inventory.

MAGICAL LEEK SOUP (BROTH)

Serves 1 for the weekend

INGREDIENTS

2 pounds leeks

1. Clean the leeks and rinse well to get rid of sand and soil. Cut off the ends of the dark green parts, leaving all the white parts plus a suggestion of pale green. (Reserve the extra greens for soup stock.)

2. Put the leeks in a large pot and cover with water. Bring to a boil, reduce the heat, and simmer uncovered for 20 to 30 minutes. Pour off the liquid and reserve. Place the leeks in a bowl.

. . . .

The juice is to be drunk (reheated or at room temperature to taste) every 2 to 3 hours, 1 cup at a time.

For meals, or whenever hungry, have some of the leeks themselves, ½ cup at a time. Drizzle with a few drops of extra-virgin olive oil and lemon juice. Season sparingly with salt and pepper. Sprinkle with chopped parsley if you wish.

This will be your nourishment for both days, until Sunday dinner, when you can have a small piece of meat or fish (4 to 6 ounces—don't lose that scale yet!), with 2 vegetables, steamed with a bit of butter or olive oil, and a piece of fruit.

Pity those who don't love the sweet taste and delicate texture of leeks. Eventually, you probably will. If not, follow the example of my cousin in Aix-en-Provence; after the birth of two sons, she needed to shed a few pounds but didn't love leeks. A neighbor suggested hiding the leeks among other flavorful and healthful ingredients. This Provençal version is known as *soupe mimosa* (Mimosa Soup).

MIMOSA SOUP

Serves 1 for the weekend

1. Clean and chop all vegetables in rough pieces and put them in a pot, except for the cauliflower and parsley. Cover with water, bring to a boil, and simmer, uncovered, for 40 minutes. Add the cauliflower and cook for another 15 minutes.

2. Pass all the cooked vegetables through a food mill.

3. Serve the soup in a bowl and add parsley and pieces of chopped hard-boiled eggs.

INGREDIENTS

1 head lettuce
½ pound carrots
½ pound celeriac
½ pound turnips
1 pound leeks
½ pound cauliflower
½ cup chopped parsley
2 hard-boiled eggs, chopped

. . . .

Eat 1 cup (at room temperature or reheated) every 3 hours or so all day Saturday and Sunday until Sunday dinner when you can have a small piece (4 to 6 ounces) of fish or meat, 2 steamed vegetables with a dash of butter or olive oil, and 1 piece of fruit. Somewhat less liquidy and magical than the leek soup, this soup is nevertheless an effective and tasty alternative.

Both versions are so good, and such an adventure for most palates, that you will have a hard time seeing them as prison rations. Especially if these tastes are new to you, jot your impressions of flavor and fragrance on the next clean page of the notebook in which you have recorded your last three weeks. In time, this exercise will intensify your pleasures, and you may want to keep a regular diary of your gastronomic experiences, including some wine notes (just as serious oenophiles do).

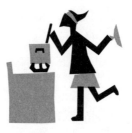

3

SHORT-TERM RECASTING: THE FIRST THREE MONTHS

While your leeks are boiling, ask yourself a couple of questions:

1. Why am I doing this? Because I'm afraid my husband or girlfriends think I am *bouboum* (overweight and dumpy)? Because none of my clothes fit? While diets are often inspired by fear and self-loathing, such emotions do not show the way toward living like a French woman. To embrace recasting, you have to be ready to embrace pleasure and individual happiness as your goals. Sounds paradoxical? At least half our bad eating and drinking habits are careless; they grow out of inattention to our true needs and delights. We don't notice what we are consuming, we

are not alert to flavors—we are not really *enjoying* our indulgences, and therefore we think nothing of them and overdo it. Perhaps you have given up caring about fashion. Or trying other new things? It may be easy for a wife, mother, and full-time worker to neglect pleasure; perhaps a part of you even thinks it's selfish. But you must understand there is nothing noble in failing to discover and cultivate your pleasures. (It will make you not only fat, but grouchy.) You owe it to your loved ones as well as yourself to know and pursue your pleasures. And since everyone's taste and metabolism are unique, you must pay attention to yourself—to what delights you—so you can tailor your system and preferences. It's a lifelong commitment, but it promises a lifetime of good health and contentment.

2. *Qu'est-ce qui se passe?* (What's going on here?) You can't start eating and living well in a physical or emotional vacuum. Why do you *think* you have gained weight? Age? Family or work pressure? Loneliness? Fashion? (Believe it or not, some of us tend to gain precisely when styles are at their least forgiving!) Just had a baby? Stopped smoking? Always hungry? Grief? Other stress? The possible combinations of mental and physical factors are too vast to list completely. Losing one's equilibrium can be a symptom of a more serious trauma. If it's a devastating problem, you may need some outside help—seek that help. But if it hasn't knocked you totally off stride, chances are you can identify and deal with it on your own. If bad eating habits are your way of compensating for another problem, stay tuned, because French women have a much more varied menu of

compensations. If you have traded in your nicotine for potato chips, it's time to consider alternatives.

Having said these things, we can proceed to plan the recasting of the next three months. First and foremost, this means identifying and reconsidering our worst offenders. Some may be eliminated, others reduced. The right approach depends on your individual needs.

"ROUND UP THE USUAL SUSPECTS"

Inspector Renault's famous line in *Casablanca,* when he lets Humphrey Bogart off the hook for killing the Nazi officer, is an apt command for the first step in recasting.

Let's look at your diary. Does anything in your past three weeks seem strange? Maybe not. Without Dr. Miracle's objective eye, I might not have immediately identified my own "offenders," those foods I was consuming out of all proportion. My big problems were bread, pastry, and chocolate. Not such rare vices. But perhaps for you they are not vices at all: your consumption of them may be perfectly moderate or trivial. One slice of bread with lunch, a small slice of tart after dinner. Your offenders may be quite different.

Analyze your diary by determining what seems excessive *in your judgment.* You might begin by asking, "What could I live without—or at least with less of?" Is the thought of those two cosmos at quitting time the only thing getting you through the day? How would *one* suit you? Or skipping every third day? Do you ask the waiter for more bread before he has even brought your order? You might find one slice savored slowly with dinner just as satisfying, or you might just as easily wait for your appetizer. Do you finish every French fry on your plate?

You see where I am going. This is not radical. Little things do add up. But now ask yourself something else: "Which things do I most enjoy: my glass of wine at dinner? an ice cream cone on Sunday afternoon?" Consider all the things you consume regularly. Which of them is giving you real pleasure and which are you having to pointless excess? One thing French women know is that the pleasure of most foods is in the first few bites; we rarely have seconds. The things we enjoy we don't enjoy as a matter of routine.

Still can't decide what to throw overboard? Okay, time to make like Inspector Renault: round up the usual suspects. Here are a few things that many women are having too much of: potato chips, bagels, pasta, pizza, fried foods, juices, beer or hard liquor, candy bars, ice cream, soda, and junky chocolate. If you have any of these daily (for instance, chips on the side whenever you have a sandwich), consider it an opportunity! If, for the next three months, you can cut out these "offenders" altogether without feeling brutalized, go for it. But if one of them is critical to your contentment, reduce incrementally. Juice diluted with sparkling water is more thirst quenching than juice straight. And you can reduce the juice part slowly. Bread is special, the staff of life for French people, not to be treated lightly. (In fact, bread, like chocolate, is one of those rare foods that can be your best friend or your worst enemy—I look closely at both in a later chapter.) But if you're having three pieces at every meal, bring it down to a piece and just pass the basket if you honestly don't want any. Do not eat on autopilot. Eventually, you will have it only when it counts!

There is a life of blissful indulgence out there with less of all these things, even the ones that are basically good for you. Getting there happens once you discover that, on the whole, "offenders" are foods we tend to eat compulsively, with less actual pleasure than you might think. Often they are poor versions of something better—for instance, supermarket processed cheeses as compared with a real cheese of real character. When you learn to replace the junk with goodies that truly satisfy, you will learn that the rule of "Less is more" is no copout. By then you'll discover what is obvious to French women: There can be an almost ecstatic enjoyment in a single piece of fine dark chocolate that a dozen Snickers bars can never give you. On that subject, please also eliminate all "chocolate" loaded with cornstarch, corn syrup, artificial flavors, artificial coloring, and too much sugar.

The great seventeenth-century philosopher Descartes is famed for his dictum "I think, therefore I am." But he also knew a thing or two about how the body and the mind influence each other and that in order to understand the passions of the soul, its functions must be distinguished from those of the body. A French woman's secret is mainly in her head. It is one thing to identify your offenders, quite another thing to manage them. If we all had an iron will, there would be no need for this book. On average, a French woman is no more likely than anyone else to possess one. But she is much likelier to have mastered the useful art of self-deception—the mental part of living well. (In fact, I'd say that complete control of the mind over the body is undesirable; it suggests a lack of openness to the spontaneous delights of the senses.) So how are ordinary mortal women to get through three months of "offender" reduction as we pursue new habits and new balance? Here are the basic principles as learned from Dr. Miracle and adjusted by trial and error over the years. They are presented initially in brief to start you on recasting, but for a lifetime subscription to the secrets of French women, you'll have to absorb them in the chapters ahead. There are more particular lessons one must learn or relearn to reconcile with food. But for now:

Slow and Steady

There is no lasting glory in rapid weight loss. That's what diets offer: a fast (weeks, not months) round of misery for temporary results. If you believe you can shed pounds quickly by force of will and deprivation, you will in all likelihood not only regain the ones you have lost, but add a few more besides. (This is the origin of the expression *yo-yo dieting*.) If your recasting starts showing dramatic results within a month, you are among the lucky. But a proper recasting, resetting your body's dials, is a three-month affair. The key is to make it a pleasant three months, not a sentence in the Bastille.

Variety

As Dr. Miracle counseled, crash diets also run the risk of creating *carences* (nutritional deficiencies), the dangers of which can be worse than those of excess weight. The answer is not in supplements, but in eating the greatest possible variety of good foods. Such variety will go a long way toward compensating you for those things you miss—you will actually find yourself not missing them so much.

It's amazing to French women how much of the same old things some people will eat. Gastronomic boredom leads to lots of unhealthy eating. If you don't make improvisation and experimentation part of your eating life, you are sure to find yourself in an eating rut. It's as bad as a romantic rut—losing that spark—and just as likely to get you in trouble! French women know the importance of turning a bit of comfort into excitement. Don't know your way around the market? Don't have time to cook? Relax: you don't have to be rich or a three-star chef to enjoy a vast world of natural flavors. Once you learn a few tricks, it takes surprisingly little effort to cook with variety and no more time than Monday night meat loaf. (The next chapter has some examples, and there is a complete arsenal in "The Seasons and the Seasonings.")

Consider this an opportunity to try foods and flavors you have never tried before. A new cheese you've heard of? A fresh herb? What about skate or shallots or mâche or celery root? Or any number of varieties of oyster, one of my personal favorites. Novelty is a powerful distraction. Choose quality over quantity: pick things in season. Usually the best in season is cheaper than the worst off-season!

A final trick of variety: Since the pleasure of most foods is in the first few bites, eat one thing on your plate at a time, at least at the start of the meal when you can concentrate and enjoy the full flavors. The mouthful as mélange (blend of foods) defeats the purpose of variety.

Ritual Preparation

French women love to shop and prepare food. They love to talk about what they have bought and made. It's a deeply natural love, but one that is erased in many other cultures. Most French women learn it from their mothers, some from their fathers. But if your parents aren't French, you can still learn it yourself. Even though I was a student, Dr. Miracle sent me to one of the best local markets in the rue Clerc, near where I lived in Paris, two to three times a week. His advice was simple: Buy only what you need for the next day or two. (Forget your twice-a-month megahauls from the supermarket.) I was to cook simply but cook at home so as to see and learn what I was putting into my body. In recasting, it is a great help to make and bring your own lunch. Avoid the unknowns of prepared foods, especially the processed kind. (Easier than bringing your scale to work!) It was equally important to transform my evening meal into a sort of "gourmand" happening. "What's for dinner?" was to become an exciting question with varied answers. Thought and preparation must go into your supper. You must decide that the results you want are worth a little extra thought and effort in the beginning. In no time you will find yourself doing it automatically. Marketing and cooking were relatively new to me—I somehow hadn't picked up much about them at home, though there were great cooks in my family—but Dr. Miracle insisted that I would have fun with it. Fortunately, most of my university classes didn't start until late morning.

Water

Everyone, French and non-French, agrees it is critical and most of us don't get enough. But it is certainly a boring prospect to gulp down eight glasses a day as needed. And while many women make a fetish of carrying a water bottle around with them all day, I wonder how many are getting all they need. However much you're having, more can't hurt. If you can't think of reaching eight glasses a day, for now add two as follows: Have one big glass first thing in the morning. Few of us realize how dehydrating our sleep time can be. (Perhaps this is one reason why a huge glass of juice—an offender by any standard—seems so good first thing.) A morning glass will not only freshen your complexion, it will help perk you up if you haven't slept well. And have a glass when you go to sleep at night. Dehydration is one cause of bad sleep. If you don't have a taste for water, try slicing a lemon into your glass.

Ritual Eating

A whole section on this later. For now, basic survival skills: Eat only at the table, only sitting down. Never eat out of cartons. Use real plates and decent napkins, if you have them, to emphasize the seriousness of the activity. Eat slowly, chew properly. (American mothers tell you this but tend to see it as a matter of politeness rather than pleasure.) Do not watch television or read the paper. Think only about what you are eating, smelling and savoring every bite. Practice putting down your utensils between every few bites, describing to yourself the flavors and textures in your mouth. (Don't let anyone mock you for acting like a French woman—you will laugh last!)

Portion Control

Learn it slowly. Portion size has been a losing battle for Americans, a gastronomic Waterloo, in fact. Cut back gently, especially if your problem is too much of a good thing. Salmon is wonderful health food, but if you need half a pound to feel content, you need too much. Keep the scale handy and reduce ounce by ounce, until four to six ounces seems a satisfying amount to you. This point reveals a key grotesquerie of the protein diet: You can stuff yourself silly with bacon as long as bread doesn't pass your lips. (Utterly *dégueulasse!*) As a rule, half a pound of anything in one sitting is too much. You won't even notice the change in satisfaction, but the bodily change will astound you.

Don't Stock the Offenders

Some foods we eat automatically in whatever quantity we have on hand. Can't be content with just a handful of nuts? Don't keep them in the house! Very few of us will go out just to buy a bag of salty nuts or potato chips. If you have them, and keep going back for more, try to apply the preceding principle of progressive downsizing. If your first handful is six, make that the limit. The next time consider stopping at three for the day.

Substitution and Pacifiers

Knowing my biggest problem was sweets, Dr. Miracle furnished a recipe that provided much of the satisfaction at a fraction of the calories. Like all his best prescriptions, it has remained useful ever since.

APPLE TART WITHOUT DOUGH

Serves 4

The following recipe for an apple tart without a crust is less sweet—lower in calories—but more nutritional than what one finds in pastry shops, delis, or supermarkets. Homemade versus prepared food: a universe of difference. Read labels and start avoiding foods whose ingredients sound like chemical weapons.

INGREDIENTS

4 medium-size Golden
Delicious apples
2 tablespoons lemon juice
4 cabbage leaves
1 tablespoon sugar
¼ teaspoon cinnamon
Dots of butter

1. Peel and core the apples, cut into quarters, slice each quarter into thirds, and sprinkle with the lemon juice. Place the apples on the cabbage leaves, shaping the slices like those on a small tart.

2. Preheat the oven to 275 degrees. Mix the sugar with the cinnamon and sprinkle almost all of it on the apple slices (leaving enough to cover the dots of butter). Add small dots of butter and cover with the remaining sugar-cinnamon mixture. Bake the tart in the preheated oven for 15 minutes. Serve warm or at room temperature.

· · · · · · · · · · · · · · ·

You don't need to eat the cabbage leaves, though you can; they are for presentation and don't affect the tart. And yes, after your three months, you can go back to having a slice of the real thing with a *pâte brisée* crust.

Discretion is often the better part of valor. Dr. Miracle proposed I avoid troublemakers, in my case sweets, as a child is taught to walk away from a fight. It would be better, he said, if at the beginning I went to school without money, or no more than I would need for the Métro or to buy a cup of coffee. For me, avoidance of the pastry shops also meant varying my route. If you walk to work, don't go the same way every day; variety is important in environment as well as in nutrition. Dr. Miracle knew Paris well and would test me on all the monuments, public squares, and buildings where famous people lived (Gertrude Stein on rue de Fleurus or Edith Wharton on rue de l'Université). I found myself entering the porte cochere of every beautiful *hôtel particulier* on my route to the Sorbonne. No one in my family had been to Paris for more than a brief visit, so they were intrigued as I fell in love with the great city.

If your offenders are not lurking in the streets, or your streets are not so compelling, try to stimulate your other senses. One thing drawing me into the patisseries was the heavenly smell of baked goods. Buying some fragrant flowers was not only a treat, but a defense. I'd sniff them when I came near a bakery. Since smell is half of taste, it's hard to crave sweets when you don't smell them. A sachet of fragrant lavender can also do wonders.

Move

Perhaps you live in a place where driving is the norm. Or perhaps you don't have occasion to walk every day. That does not change the fact that your weight is determined by two variables: what you consume and what you burn off. Dr. Miracle knew I didn't like sports (most French women don't), but I still needed to *me remuer* (move my butt). A twice-a-day twenty-minute walk to school was the perfect remedy for me. If you live too far from work or school to walk, try walking part of the way. Or take a half-hour walk at lunch or after dinner. A walk not only uses calories, it can be wonderfully meditative, clearing your head and making you less vulnerable to eating for psychological comfort. The key is to add moderately to your daily physical exertion. If you use an elevator, try taking the stairs instead; over the course of a week the added calories are significant, but the added trouble is minimal.

"Never Be Hungry"

One of Dr. Miracle's wisest prescriptions, it is especially important in the first weeks of recasting as your body is learning the new world order. Hunger is distracting and unpleasant, almost as much as being bloated or stuffed. You should no more skip meals than you would skip filling your gas tank— you'll only be stranded later. Our aim is not to challenge the laws of physics. Feed it reasonably and on schedule and your body's engine is less likely to answer you with screaming hunger. Strict attention to this principle is key until the mind has been tamed. One vital secret of hunger management Dr. Miracle taught me is yogurt—not the sugary supermarket kind, but the real stuff, strained, which is not only of superior texture and flavor, but full of the bacteria essential to health. It isn't readily available in America, unless you live near a dairy. But you can make it yourself once a week according to an

incredibly easy recipe. Dr. Miracle prescribed two small servings a day during recasting, to be had as I wished: with breakfast, as a dessert, or for a snack. A little honey or wheat germ
or fresh fruit made it seem more like a treat, but when I developed a taste for it, I began to love it *plain,* for its silky, creamy
tartness. A yogurt eaten just when I knew hunger would strike
was a terrific pacifier. (See recipe on page 151.)

En-Cas

We also had to have some provision for off-site emergencies.
Dr. Miracle explained what he called my *en-cas* (literally, "in
case" . . . of hunger attack). It was so simple: Always have a
little something in your pocket, something your body will register as a *minirepas* (snack). It's not only handy, but a powerful
psychological deterrent. It shuts up my *petits démons.* Knowing
it was there made me less anxious, less likely to crave. When I
did break out the *en-cas,* enjoying it left me less hungry at dinnertime. Compensation. I still carry it: a small bag of soy nuts,
which nowadays often appears when my flight is delayed. It
should be something good for you but satisfying.

Weekend Rewards

Dr. Miracle understood only too well that we are fragile
beings in a world full of temptations. Deprivation is the
mother of failure. Any program that your mind interprets as
punishment is one your mind is bound to rebel against.
Whether your pleasure is a glass of wine with dinner or a
croissant for breakfast, you simply cannot deprive yourself for
extended periods of time and not expect your body to take
revenge. So even during recasting, your body needs a Sab-

bath. Mind you, we are not talking about an all-you-can-eat bender, during which you consume everything you managed to abstain from all week. Rather, this is a day of rest when you can enjoy a civilized share of some favorites. Some diet authorities advise you not to reward yourself with food, but I say it's okay as long as the food *is* rewarding: no junk, good quality, and respectfully savored.

Dr. Miracle said it was better to stray on Saturday and go back to the plan on Sunday in order to start the new week on the right track. And it made sense in my case. While I was a student, I was often invited for Saturday supper at the home of some rather fancy friends in Paris. They had a full-time cook—an extraordinary luxury anywhere—whose elaborate offerings made it difficult to pick among my vices. (You can see why I held on to these friends!) Dr. Miracle's answer: *"Mais, Mireille, fais preuve d'intelligence"* ("Just use your head"). If a glass of Champagne as aperitif and a dessert seem too good to resist, have them, but then don't eat bread. Making choices that are meaningful to you is the essence of the French woman's secret.

During this phase of recasting, I was especially worried about going home for Easter in a few weeks and facing an elaborate holiday feast with my family, who were naturally less discreet than my fancy friends in Paris. I was already on the right track, and having lost about nine pounds, I didn't want to draw attention to myself or to any change in eating habits. Dr. Miracle rightly advised that nobody would notice if I ate my foie gras, skimped on most of the various breads, helped myself to just a few French fries, and enjoyed dessert. The next day, you'll compensate, he said very matter-of-factly.

He was telling me to be the master of my pleasures as well as my restraint.

Still, I had a lingering question about where this was going in the long run. Alas, it was those demon offenders again. I knew I could keep them on this short leash for only so long. When could I reintegrate them into the school week without bringing on my downfall? True, I wasn't suffering, but the good doctor had promised a life of more indulgence. And I was of the irrepressible generation of May 1968, whose rebellious slogan was *"Il est interdit d'interdire"* ("It is forbidden to forbid").

The answer, I would learn, was in the words *petit* and *peu,* which both mean "little." You can have *de tout un peu et de peu pas beaucoup,* meaning you can have a little of everything, but in small portions. As I was proud of my results, but beginning to feel slightly underprivileged, Dr. Miracle made a minor adjustment: twice a week at lunch—which was normally at a sidewalk café with friends who, like me, couldn't handle the food of the *restaurant universitaire* (the school cafeteria)—I could eat the little piece of dark chocolate (*un palet* or *carré*) that came with my espresso. I could pick the days, but not go over twice a week. Learn to pick your moments. After a hard test in the morning, I needed it. Ditto after declamation exercise in front of the class! It was a minor adjustment that gave me a big psychological lift. And it was my first peek at the power of slight recalibration. Little changes can make big differences in the long run.

Zipper Syndrome

By Easter, my recasting was complete. And I felt new things had become natural. Even now I don't recall it as a savorless time of deprivation. But what had I accomplished? What can you expect to accomplish? I was down about twelve pounds, half of what I needed to lose. *Mais attention*—I wasn't getting on the scale every day to track my progress. Scales are not a universal fixture of French bathrooms as they are in America. And they can be dispiriting indicators of progress. A woman gains weight with water retention during part of the month. Our weight can vary for other reasons, too (time of day, for instance), that have little to do with whether or not we are eating in balance. I did confirm the loss of kilos from time to time, but mainly I learned to be more attentive to the look and feel of my body in my clothes. I could see it was changing. And when the scale registered my loss of twelve pounds, it was only confirming what I seemed to know. I still find getting into some slim-cut pants the best indication of pounds melting— much easier, more reliable, and sexier. Use what French women call *le syndrome de la fermeture éclair* (zipper syndrome), or use a measuring tape.

Your equilibrium weight, as we have said, is very personal, depending on many factors, like age, body type, and for some people even time of year. Likewise, improvements are relative, not absolute. Just as French women do not count calories, they mainly do not count pounds. You will have a sense after three months of recasting how far you have yet to go. If you feel you have met about half your goal, your recast has succeeded. If not, consider how far you are and continue for a few more weeks. Be wary of unrealistic goals—we can't all be model thin. Look for a few more trade-offs: a further reduction of some offenders (guaranteed to be easier once you've already done it); an additional ten minutes of walking a day. Adjusting by small amounts is always the key to moving to your equilibrium.

To empower this lifestyle fully requires that you embrace the rule of quality over quantity. Learning to cultivate quality is what we'll consider in the chapters ahead as we take up stabilization—a time when, remarkably, you will be enjoying more pleasures and still be losing weight. First, however, let's see recasting at work for a few American women I know.

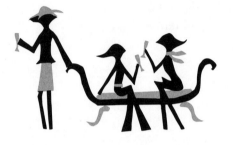

4

Let's revisit some of the basic principles of recasting:

- Look at your three-week profile; identify and reduce the "offenders" as much as you can without inducing shock. Whatever you can cut out completely without agony, just cut. Reduce others *peu à peu* (little by little).
- Eat at regular times.
- Look at portions of nonoffender foods and trim these gradually, too.
- Get to know the market, not the supermarket. Shop for food several times a week (on a need-to-eat basis, but never when hungry).
- Diversify your foods with an eye to seasons. Increase the proportion of fresh fruits and vegetables.

- Introduce and experiment with a couple of new flavors.
- Prepare your own meals. Shun prepared foods, especially processed ones with artificial anything.
- Have a real breakfast.
- Eat slowly, sitting down. Chew well, even if it seems theatrical at first.
- Introduce two daily servings of homemade (or all-natural plain) yogurt as a dessert, breakfast, or snack food.
- Drink at least two more glasses of water per day, slipping in more as you find opportunity.
- Introduce a small but regular new physical movement, a daily walk or climbing stairs. (If you go to a gym, you're probably doing enough in spandex, so pick something you can do in street clothes.)
- Don't stock offenders at home.
- Develop a list and stock of food pacifiers, substitutes for offenders.
- Keep your *en-cas* in your pocket for off-site emergencies.
- Choose and enjoy your weekend rewards.

As I say, this is not radical. But to some it may still seem a little abstract at this point (the tendency toward abstraction is admittedly a French weakness), so let's see recasting in action. Let me introduce some friends, the three Cs.

CAMILLE

Camille, thirty-five, had been fighting her weight all her life. Obese she was not, but at her height (five feet two), those extra twenty-five pounds were obvious; she felt and looked chubby. At one time or another, she had tried every diet to come along. In the end, by her own analysis, the problem was simply genetic: being overweight ran in the family. Her mother in particular had always been heavy. So deep down, Camille believed her attempts to lose weight were doomed.

Camille joined Clicquot when we acquired another firm; she brought some excellent business skills and experience. The corporate world, however, can be brutal and unfair, especially the luxury goods business, in which image is critical. In all corporations, appearance counts a lot more for women than for men. Camille's job involved regular cross-country travel, including dinners with clients. She'd been with us for a year when it became obvious that her first New York winter had not been an easy adjustment. Bulky cold-weather clothes had hidden some excesses, but once spring came around, I sensed a panic setting in, as the next round of heavy travel and entertaining loomed. We had developed a nice rapport, and one day, when I asked her how it was going, she opened up to me. I told her about my own weight calamity as a young adult and how I was able to reverse it with some simple changes. She agreed to record her consumption for three weeks.

I don't recommend jumping the gun, but it took only a glance at the first week's entries to spot some major offenders. First there was beer. It seems Camille "got thirsty" every evening, whether at home or out of town. So she would have a bottle of beer, often around eleven p.m. Drinking beer late at night seemed odd to me, especially in someone who was having wine with meals in restaurants. Could Camille have a drinking problem? No, her alcohol consumption wasn't that excessive, and she gave no other indication of such a problem.

I asked how long this nightly beer thing had been going on. Apparently since college: she would buy salty snack foods from a machine while studying and wash them down at bedtime with a beer. After giving it some thought, she admitted she didn't really love it; it was just habit, and she was just "thirsty." It was clear she had unthinkingly imported an old college habit into her adult life and retained it for fifteen years! Always one to try the obvious first, I said, "If you're thirsty, why not drink water and then go to bed?" This seemed a no-brainer that could be worth between five and ten pounds over some months if she would just recognize and tame this one offender. But it wasn't that easy. She wasn't madly craving the buzz or flavor of beer, but she did want something more interesting than water. Surprisingly, the solution for her was herbal teas. Her favorites became verbena and fresh mint, both soothing substitutes for the mildly sedative effect of bedtime beer. She was also eager to try new ones and became rather a connoisseur of teas. It took her longer to embrace drinking more plain old water during the day—key to reducing night thirst. So I suggested she just make a point of having a little paper cupful whenever she passed the cooler. When the effects began to show, she passed it more regularly.

Another problem came from business. Not only was she eating airplane food (sort of a contradiction in terms, really), but she was eating it *in addition* to having dinner on the town. Apparently whatever the flight attendants put in front of her— stale nuts, mystery meats, cloying desserts—she would eat (know anyone like this?), even with a business dinner or lunch scheduled shortly after landing. This was a relatively easy offender to banish. She knew that plane food was horrible.

Was she eating out of boredom? To pass the time? Anyway, I counseled her to have a small sandwich before boarding and to carry a bottle of chilled herbal tea she would brew the night before. Sipping it throughout the flight, as she listened to her own CDs (not piped-in music), she passed the time contentedly; she was even able to nap on board for the first time in her life. (I do it, too: whatever your seat assignment, the key is pushing liquids in the parched cabin air, which is good for hair frizz but little else.)

Her third offender was a bit more complicated. A couple of times a week, especially on weekends, she would have a huge dish of pasta as her dinner. She said it seemed to her the easiest thing one could make and still have the comfort of home cooking. This was the voice of inexperience. Obviously there were other ways of warding off the Sunday night blues. This problem called for a dramatic approach—no pasta at home for a while. But that meant finding things to cook that were equally satisfying and easy. As it was spring, the outdoor markets in New York City were a godsend. I showed her simple, delicious ways of cooking beets, fennel, broccoli, and carrots with accents like chopped herbs and lemon juice. The flavors of fresh vegetables in season dazzled her. Anyone who has ever had a farm-fresh tomato will attest that with a little salt and olive oil, plus some chopped parsley or basil, that alone can seem like a meal. Making choices at her own pace, and to her own taste, she found it wonderfully easy to increase her fruits and vegetables. Following a simple recipe for fish (page 99)—which, as a kitchen novice, she had never even attempted—she was enjoying at home a meal that would have seemed luxurious by most restaurant standards. She also found twenty minutes to walk each day (from the office after work, as she was not a morning person). She would ordinarily have had one transfer, but she took the subway to the transfer point and walked home from there.

After three months she'd lost ten pounds. On a small frame, it showed big-time. And as she liked the changes she had made, she seemed in no imminent danger of gaining it back. In fact, she was eager to experiment with new ways of painlessly losing the rest. I noticed some new clothes, a self-confidence I had not seen before, and a happier face. Others noticed, too.

CAROLINE

Caroline was a generation older and someone I met at a seminar for women business leaders. Most of her life she had had no breakfast except a cigarette or two and a cup of coffee with double sugar. This, again, seemed like a college girl's habit, though Caroline's college days were long behind her. Now that she had quit smoking for good—after many failed attempts—she was starving in the morning. She had gained ten pounds over the past year and seemed prepared to accept it, though crankily, as the inevitable trade-off for not smoking. Her nonsmoker's breakfast was not much of an improvement: a glass of orange juice from the carton (a hit of pure sugar), two cups of coffee with two or more teaspoons of sugar each (sugar with coffee, really), and two biscotti (more sugar). Not only too sweet, but boring. Her diary also revealed a taste for dishes with heavy sauces, odd, given the relatively mild weather.

The rest of her eating pattern wasn't too bad, though she suffered from the extremely common problems of not enough vegetables, fruit, or water. Her principal offender was sugar in various forms, plain and hidden. She could never skip dessert, to which weakness I could easily relate. Less typical was her love of cheese. Having traveled a bit with her husband, she had a keen sense of quality, favoring some that might seem too pungent for the average American. (Offenders can't be too personal.) But she hadn't learned what a proper portion is. Here is where a little scale comes in handy: three ounces is a lot better than eight.

Changing breakfast wasn't easy. Some of us can't quite start the day without coffee and cannot drink coffee without sugar. Often, though, this comes from drinking bad coffee: instant, freeze-dried, or reheated. Fewer need sugar given the taste of freshly ground coffee, though it still can take a bit of an adjustment. With a cheap little coffee grinder, it took only thirty extra seconds to brew a luxurious, aromatic pot; and Caroline was able to reduce the sweetening progressively to half a teaspoon by the third week. She eliminated the orange juice gradually—a third at a time over three weeks—replacing it with a fruit later in the day. The biscotti gave way to a slice of whole-grain bread with a sliver of butter. (People who would never dream of butter at breakfast don't understand what a luxury the smallest amount can seem.) And to give it some heft that would hold her till lunch, we added yogurt, at first with a little drizzle of the acacia honey I had put her on to, but soon unsweetened. Sure enough, she was seeing breakfast now not as a sugar-charged jump start, but as a ritual of self-pampering; it put her in a sunnier mood to face the day.

Dessert in restaurants was a challenge. Like many empty-nest New Yorkers, she and her husband often ate out in the neighborhood for convenience' sake, and there was always a sweet temptation among the specials. Fortunately it was summer, and fresh berries, melons, and figs didn't seem a hardship, particularly when served with good yogurt—as they were at her local Greek restaurant. But when some baked or gooey confection beckoned, there was no need to fight it. Order one dessert and slowly savor one or two forkfuls. The rest she could pass on to her husband or friends: "Let *them* eat cake."

The attraction to heavy sauces was weird. Actually, an old friend explained it to me when I noticed his preference for them while eating out in Paris. Smoking wreaks havoc on the olfactory mucous membranes, and these are slow to repair themselves even after we quit. Since aromas are more soluble in fatty dishes, taste buds naturally find such fare more satisfying when the smelling component of taste has been a bit incapacitated. So as not to deprive her of flavor, it was important then to reduce these fatty dishes ever so slowly for a while, and Caroline complied once she understood the problem. The nose also explained her overindulgence with pungent cheeses. When one is dining at someone's home in France, the cheese course is the only one that may be politely refused. This was too polite for Caroline's taste, however, so she started cutting back, little by little. She also started cooking with more pungent flavors—turmeric, curry, hot peppers—harder for her palate or her recovering nose to miss. In time, milder flavors would begin to register again.

Caroline took to walking the six floors up to and down

from her apartment whenever she had nothing to carry and taking a twenty-minute walk three times a week. She had no trouble learning to move like a typical French woman. Eleven pounds came off in ten weeks, and she had to allow that far from feeling deprived, she felt more self-indulgent than she could ever remember. Do her changes seem like deprivation to you?

CONNIE

Connie's case was a bit more complicated. She was in her early twenties and very much unaware of what she was eating. She had grown up in the suburban Midwest, where food shopping was a twice monthly affair, when her mother would load the fridge, the pantry, and especially the freezer with provisions for the next two weeks. Foodstuffs were just other items on a shopping list that included toilet paper and soap. On her own, Connie was buying the same brands of frozen entrées that were her mother's tried-and-true. Home-cooked dinner back home had been a Sunday ritual, the only meal shared *en famille.* During the week, everyone ate according to his or her busy schedule (both parents are lawyers). Connie's mother had a handful of recipes she used again and again. They represented the comforts of home, so they became the only things Connie ever attempted to cook when she entertained friends in her studio walk-up. Otherwise, she had an unapologetic love of some all-American staples: burgers, pizza, cheddar cheese, Stouffer's lasagna. Supermarket cookies and pints of ice cream were always on hand, but nary a fresh vegetable or fruit. The drinks were soda, *encore* soda, *toujours* soda. Not a pretty scenario. The fridge was packed with giant-size soda bottles, both regular and diet. So when she wasn't pouring sugar into her body, she was imbibing an awful concoction of chemicals.

When we met she was starting her career in New York and for the first time trying desperately to lose weight—a good fifteen pounds. Oddly, she didn't feel so overweight in college-girl clothes, which, as one may notice, have been much more revealing in the past five years. But in more demure professional attire, she never felt soignée (my word, admittedly; I can't remember hers). I got to know her working on a project with another firm, and when I took her out to lunch, she watched me with obvious puzzlement as I ate everything and sipped a glass of Veuve Clicquot. When they brought the coffee, she said rather sweetly, "May I ask you a very personal question?" I knew what was coming and encouraged her to dish. Like many young women, she had tried lots of deprivation diets without lasting success. On her last venture, a strict no-carb affair, she had eaten unprecedented portions of eggs, bacon, and cheese—some of her favorites. Finally, she would go off whatever diet it was, and without fail, the only lasting result was a bigger appetite for the things the diet had allowed her to have. She had also tried and failed to burn off weight through punishing workouts. Someone had told her that if she spent one hour a day on some machine, her eating habits wouldn't matter. Connie had just bought a three-month membership to a gym with every cent she wasn't spending on her New York rent. I never fail to marvel at the willingness of Americans to pound away at a StairMaster for hours rather than make a few relatively painless adjustments. Connie had lost a couple of pounds, but her daily machine regimen was like working on a chain gang, and she quit after a few weeks, subsequently gaining the weight back.

I suggested she continue going to the gym, since she had paid for it and would probably hate herself for bagging it altogether. But I counseled moderation: a half hour of something aerobic three times a week, no more, and not the same three things every week. She would also have to change some of her eating habits ASAP. As it was the dead of winter, the Magical Leek Soup kickoff seemed absolutely de rigueur. It would be tougher on someone who lived on her kind of food, I thought, but it would be good for her morale to get a quick start. By the following Monday morning, she had achieved what had taken two weeks of forced labor at the gym. Two pounds—mostly water, true, but nevertheless two pounds—were gone. It was indeed a boost to her spirits, but something even more remarkable happened: she had discovered a new pleasure. "I can't believe how delicious leeks are! I just love them!" she told me. Even I was a bit surprised. In fact, long after her first weekend of eating like a French woman, Connie would from time to time gladly have leek soup for lunch.

Connie described her first three months as almost effortless, practically entertaining. The kind of cooking I introduced her to was a deliciously diverting novelty. Winter is a wonderful time for hearty fare, and she especially enjoyed the luxury of my easy Chicken au Champagne (page 176). But the fruits and vegetables are also great: she loved to poach pears—couldn't believe a fat-free dessert you can make in eight to ten minutes could be this good! (Just place pears in a pot of boiling water with red wine and a touch of cinnamon and sugar and let cool. See page 143 for a recipe.) She even served it to friends, who went gaga. Because her diet had been as bland and fattening as any I've seen, the substitutions she made were quick to take effect. According to the rules, she never allowed herself to be hungry; for maximum satisfaction, we tried to confine the high-fat foods to snacks—nutritious and satisfying handfuls of nuts and small cubes of cheese. As for her new adventures in the kitchen, these were much lower in fat but much higher in previously unfamiliar flavors (anise, hazelnut oil instead of olive oil on mesclun). And so, lucky girl, she didn't even miss burgers and pizza. She still had them once or twice a week when eating out, but with her growing awareness of possibilities, they began to seem too dull to eat more often. And in time, the portion control even of those varied offenders was automatic. After a month, two slices of pizza for lunch, formerly her "usual," just seemed too heavy and greasy. Her diet sodas were no asset, but not an immediate problem, either. I let her wean herself off them, replacing them with a little fresh fruit juice diluted with seltzer. (Sometimes it's healthier overall to add a few calories for the sake of quality.)

Connie was fortunate in terms of how easily she could switch off her offenders and make substitutions. Her case shows the importance of assessing yourself as an individual rather than following a diet. Each of us has strengths and weaknesses. What is relatively easy for you may be hard for someone else, and vice versa. And of course, what tickles your fancy may not tickle another's as much, or as we say in French, *à chacun son goût!* (to each his or her taste).

One thing that really tickled Connie as she developed her

sense of food was presentation. Over the summer she had worked for a very fancy caterer, whose creations for weddings and other events had to be not just delicious, but gorgeous to behold. The attention to detail appealed to Connie's meticulous personality, and it opened her eyes to what the French mean by the word *menu*—not just a list of options, but a selection of little dishes. The order of food, the arrangement of food on the plate, can often dramatically affect our experience, especially our sense of a proper portion. A tuna carpaccio artfully formed can be much more satisfying to eat than the same amount scattered on a plate like the dog's supper. This is part of *les rites de la table* I discuss in the following chapter.

After her first three weeks, Connie had lost four pounds and was already full of new energy. Her mood had changed, too. Four pounds on the average woman's frame is significant, and she felt herself starting to slide in her clothes. She immediately wanted to buy something in the next size down, but I convinced her to wait. If experience was any indication, she'd be down another size before long.

ET ALORS?: GETTING STARTED

Three examples do hardly a recipe for success make. But that is the point: in this strategy for weight loss and wellness *à la française*, there are no recipes, only ingredients. As with good cooking, the result will depend on what you use and what pleases you. There are some elements that apply to all cases: a little more walking, a little more water, for instance. But otherwise the approach is unapologetically individualist and will depend somewhat on trial and error. The key is to cultivate your own intuition of your offenders and pleasures and adjust each accordingly by degrees that suit you. (Consider it your vote for the Franco-American ideal of individual liberty over the tyrannical regime of one-size diets.) For this reason, three months is the usual time to find your way. But you must enjoy the ride. Three months of hard-core dieting might well be enough to crush any woman's spirit, but three months of discovering new things and getting to know your body better is a kindness to yourself that will continue to be repaid for years to come.

We have not and will not be judging our successes by obsessive attention to calories, carbohydrates, proteins, fats, lipids, glucose, or other chemical structures or units. Most French women are not like Madame Curie and would be bored to tears reading about such things, much less applying them to one of the most sacred parts of life, food. Remember to tiptoe onto the bathroom scale only once in a while, but not daily. Judge your progress by your eyes and hands, using your clothes and your mirror as guides. And use the food scale to get to know one- to five-ounce portions whether it's fish, meat, or dessert, particularly pie and cake!

Approaching your equilibrium weight (*bien dans ta peau*) is a natural and intuitive progression, a course of fine-tuning that embraces both discovery and moderation.

I am happy to report that years later Connie looks terrific and ready for the pages of *Vogue.* Caroline has maintained her equilibrium, perhaps a couple of pounds below the set point I would have picked for her, but she's happy. And Camille? I've lost track of her and have often wondered. Of the three, she was the least happy to begin with, too reliant on food as therapy and heredity as an excuse. But if she has maintained her new optimism, I'd bet she's fine now.

Having read to this point, you should have enough strategies to start recasting, but we have plenty more in stock. *Allons-y!*

Manger bien et juste
(Eat well and eat right)
—Molière

Your three months should bring you at least halfway toward your target equilibrium weight, even further if your recasting goals are modest. Again, you should pay attention to yourself, your eyes, complexion, state of mind, and, above all, clothes— these will tell you where you are. If you are there—and only you can tell for sure—brava! You are ready for stabilization. If you feel you are not yet halfway, however, you should extend your recasting as you see fit. A good dressmaker will always require you to come in for several fittings; with each, the alterations become more subtle. If you continue to recast, see where you might be prepared to "take it in a little" for the sake of continued progress. But always bear in mind the golden rules: *Fais-toi plaisir* (Take your pleasures and diversions); keep reducing what you can *peu à peu*. While you may have reached some levels of consumption you would have considered unrealistic three months ago (for instance, only two slices of bread a day), your contentment may well extend into even smaller amounts (one slice). Experimentation is the only way to find out how little you need to feel satisfied.

Assuming successful recasting, you are ready to start increasing your share of the things you enjoy. You are ready for stabilization. This again is governed entirely by an understanding of your personal "cost-pleasure benefit" analysis. You may feel virtuous having stuck mainly to less fattening desserts for three months, as I did under Dr. Miracle. But now you'd like to enjoy something ultraluscious with a bit more regularity (not just on the weekend). Guess what: you've earned it! Three months of steady progress is bound to coincide with a much greater awareness of your own nutrition and appetites. You are now more familiar with what you like and why. So it's only fair and in keeping with our pleasure principle that you reward yourself. Does this necessarily mean you will stop losing weight? *Pas du tout.* If that happens, simply backtrack and do a little more incremental cutting, even have yourself a magical leek weekend, if need be, to rally the troops. But if you ramp up as carefully as you cut back, you can easily continue to slim down while enjoying more of what you love most. "The only way to get rid of a temptation is to yield to it," observed Oscar Wilde (who died in Paris). Well, he is right to some extent. Eating is a sensual pleasure, so after the three months it's natural that we would want some more sizzle as we stabilize for life. How? It's simply a matter of taking from Peter to pay Paul. When you add an indulgence, make a corresponding reduction to compensate. Add another half hour of walking the next day. Skip the cocktail. Pass the breadbasket. Just as you've become attuned to where your greatest pleasures come from, you will also have come to know which compensations work best for you. Keep your balance week by week. French women seem to know by instinct, but as with any magic trick, it's really just a matter of practice. The key to continued weight loss is keeping one's compensations just slightly ahead of one's indulgences. This French practice of "fooling yourself" allows you to maximize your impression of pleasure, and if you do it right, voilà: the compensations will seem trivial by comparison. The net effect is a feeling of contentment and never of deprivation. Your mind must be your partner in keeping your weight at equilibrium, and as the *philosophes* would concur, you could not have a more powerful ally in this game.

But let me not journey into the abstract. The key to further progress and a lifetime of healthy eating lies in a deeper understanding of what French women know. You've had French for beginners; now it's time for the next level or two.

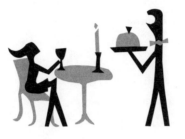

5

IL FAUT DES RITES

Saint-Exupéry's *Le Petit Prince* is a book all French people know well. It can be read in an hour but is packed with timeless wisdom. In *Le Petit Prince,* the fox explains to the little prince, *"Il faut des rites"* ("We need rituals"). As the French know well, ritual is how we give meaning to different aspects of being alive, including the most elemental: birth, marriage, death, and through it all, until the end, eating. There are, of course, holiday rituals, like the *galette des rois* eaten on the twelfth night of Christmas to commemorate the three kings. But there are also *rites quotidiens,* the rituals of everyday life by which a civilization defines itself, like *le pain quotidien,* our daily bread, or even brushing our teeth. Whether aware of it or not, we spend most of our waking hours performing our daily rituals.

In a world in which everything continues to change ever faster, these rituals are a frame of reference as well as a source of comfort and reassurance. They are also key to our well-being, part of our cultural programming about what is right and good, the norms around which we form our own tastes. Americans have some superb gastronomic rituals. Nothing French can quite compete with a hamburger barbecued on a Sunday afternoon in summer. (In fact, lots of French people adore hamburgers, as well as sirloin steaks; a few even like corn on the cob, though in France that is usually reserved for livestock.) But America is a relatively young country by European standards and, being a great nation of immigrants, much less uniform as to its gastronomic norms. While this multitude of influences has produced many delicious results, America still lags in developing the sorts of coherent principles of eating that only a thousand years of history could achieve. Even among the oldest nations of Europe, France is distinguished in the evolution of its gastronomic rituals. Where else might you be drawn into heated debates over whether the best coffee macaroons were to be found at the patisserie Ladurée or Fauchon or Pierre Hermé. The intensity still brings an impish smirk to the face of my American husband, Edward. Quality is a passion, even a compulsion.

In the late eighteenth century, as the bourgeoisie headed off the aristocracy, *les arts de la table* were born, a new code governing everything from seating arrangements to presentation to the principles of flavor harmony—our sense of what complements what. The table became a spectacle. Standard dishes received their classical names, and there followed a rush of innovation, imitation, and, indeed, fashion. Few Americans, even *Michelin*-guided gastrotourists, really appreciate the extent to which our cooking is like our couture. For all our insistence on the permanence and perfection of the classics, eating would become unbearably dull if we did not remain committed to renewing and enlivening it continually. This value has often been lost at American French restaurants, in which the same old warhorses of *cuisine bourgeoise* and the bistro are typically trotted out year after year. The French enjoy eating out in a special way, knowing that what they savor today may never again appear on the menu. They treat every meal as something special, and this is what you must learn to do, too.

Having matured over the centuries, French gastronomic culture is for the first time endangered because of globalization. With transnational fast-food outlets appearing in all our cities, it is becoming more difficult to transmit our proudly evolved values to our children. Sometimes it seems we are headed back to the Renaissance, when we ate with our fingers, helped ourselves unceremoniously from communal heaps of food, even gnawed on a bone before passing it to a neighbor. Okay, *j'exagère,* but if anything could launch a French obesity epidemic such as what has struck America, the loss of traditional values is the most likely culprit. For this reason, tradition must be honored and promoted for the betterment of all.

THREE MEALS A DAY, THREE-COURSE DINNERS

The traditional French meal is still a three-course affair, often with an additional course of cheese before the dessert. In a grand restaurant, it is not strange to have several more courses! Why don't French women, or men, for that matter, get fat? The reason is that we have adapted traditional eating to modern living, which typically includes less than traditional levels of exertion. We eat grandly on occasion, not regularly. Our courses are greater in number but smaller in size. Very important, even an ordinary meal partakes to a degree of the formality of tradition.

In the recasting section, I preached the importance of not multitasking while you eat—no TV, newspaper, or eating at the wheel or on the subway. I also suggested that some formalities can enhance the dining experience and make eating less seem more meaningful. This is the power of presentation, which includes the use of china, glassware, and table linens. Candlelight is a nice touch, too, though really an American tradition that is now all the rage in France. If the added bother strikes you as senseless extra effort, you are missing the point: setting one's table can be nearly as important as preparing the food. It focuses the mind on what lies ahead and whets the appetite, opening it to a fuller experience.

The French word *menu* not only means "bill of fare," for which *la carte* is the more common term in France, but also "little"; and by its use in relation to food, we mean to suggest our sense of small offerings. The essence of French gastronomy is to have a little of several things rather than a lot of one or two. This is the exact opposite of the American sense of portion (remember Camille's huge dish of pasta). Let us consider the French plate. It's strange to us to have a whole meal on one dish, stranger still to see any plate covered with food. The arrangement of a course in the center of the plate is part of French enjoyment. Changing plates not only compels you to concentrate on what you are enjoying at that moment, it slows the meal down, improving digestion and promoting contentment. The faster you eat, the more you'll need. If washing an extra plate seems a bother, how does it compare with getting fat?

Our *menu* servings are what allow us to enjoy now and then the full production of haute cuisine, including *amuse-bouche* (starter), first course, main course, cheese course, dessert, petits fours—the works! But mind you, these are not Louis XIV–style affairs. If the courses were not *menu,* we would never survive them. Even rising from the most elaborate meal, the French feel content, never stuffed.

Nowadays, many French still eat the main meal at lunch. This may not be practical for you. Nevertheless, three meals a day are a must to set the body's metabolism at a steady rate. Snacking, which results mainly from not having three proper meals, is generally an unhelpful expedient that confuses us, body and mind. If you are not especially hungry in the morning, don't be deceived into thinking you can get away with a faux breakfast. You'll only eat out of proportion later in the day. I've seen lots of young women who have nothing but coffee in the morning and work through lunch (if they can make it through the eleven o'clock coffee and pastry break) with an eye to an indulgent night out with friends. It might seem they are compensating earlier for pleasures to be taken later (in fact, pleasure should, as a rule, precede compensation), but in reality, the one-meal-a-day gals are only fooling themselves, and not in a good way. They are famished by dinnertime, when the party often begins with a "colored drink": hard liquor, sugary syrup (empty calories that dull the senses: these cocktails should carry the surgeon general's warning!). Then comes the typical restaurant meal, featuring oversize portions of dishes made with all the tricks of the bad chef: too much salt and fat, and sugar hidden even in the savory courses. How much? Who knows—we can't send dinner to the lab for analysis. The take-out option can be the same mystery grab bag. Save dining out for occasions and choose quality. Good restaurants are exceptional. Eat at home otherwise. *Manger bien et juste.* Know thy food and know thyself!

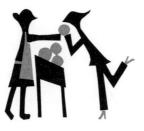

6

THE SEASONS AND THE SEASONINGS

LES FRAISES D'ANTAN:
THE STRAWBERRIES OF YESTERYEAR

There were no strawberries at the first Thanksgiving. Wild New England cranberries, perhaps. Strawberries, no. The Pilgrims naturally worked with local produce and what was in season. So did our grandparents and more remote ancestors. Tomatoes in December? Try South America. Canning and mass global distribution of produce have conditioned us to expect all foods all year round. I myself have been beguiled by the engineered good looks of off-season produce, but one taste of cardboard is enough to send me reaching for my napkin to expel the offending counterfeit. Nothing is more flavorless than a supermarket tomato in winter, but a true vine-ripened specimen in summer is nothing short of divine.

There is a reason to have pumpkin pie with Thanksgiving turkey and not with Fourth of July hot dogs. Seasonality is all about adapting your eating to what is available at markets for a short time during specific months of the year. The rhythm of the season is a vital part of tuning our bodies to their equilibrium, cultivating well-being. In summer, for example, our bodies naturally welcome a salad composed of the freshest greens, the most fragrant tomatoes; fresh corn and succulent berries delight us—each full of nutrients but also cooling water, which we lose faster in warm weather. In fall and winter, we will naturally yearn for more concentrated energy to keep warm and on the move. We want more proteins, and so happily begins the season for oysters, seafood, warm hearty soups, dried beans and lentils, and more meat.

In the end, seasonality is the key to the French woman's psychological pleasure in food—the natural pleasure of anticipation, change, the poignant joy we take in something we know we shall soon lose and cannot take for granted. Such heightened awareness of what we put in our mouths is the opposite of routine, mindless eating that promotes boredom and weight gain. The first soft-shell crabs of the season are a singular treat. The first strawberries can trigger a precious memory, as we hearken back to seasons past. And this applies to things we make as well as to produce. As I write this passage, it is Christmas Eve. From the window of our Paris apartment, we can see a famous pastry shop, Mulot, where about sixty people under umbrellas are patiently lined up in the rainy street, waiting to collect their *bûche de Noël,* the Yule log cake. Believe me, they are not annoyed to be there—*au contraire!* (Only in France, you might say, and unfortunately,

you'd be right.) The cake is rich and fattening and delicious . . . and no French woman would do without a slice or
two. Made to be eaten only a few days a year, it is a tradition
no one skips. And with a cultivated sense of balance, no one
needs to.

Whether in the French provincial villages, cities, or Paris itself,
on certain days of the week you can always see the trucks in
the local squares and lining the streets. This caravan is hauling
fresh produce, the best of the season, from meat and game to
fruits and vegetables, herbs and spices. Have you ever seen
twenty-seven varieties of olives in as many barrels? Market
day is a tradition dating back centuries, since before France
was Gaul. Why does it persist in the twenty-first century even
as French conglomerates have erected *hypermarchés* (supermarkets that could rival any American ones in size)? Why do
people of all walks of life brave the cold and heat, rain or
shine, to choose among three varieties of string beans, seven
types of potatoes, various shapes of bread, quail eggs, organic
hens, wild boar, forty-three varieties of cheese, untold num-
bers of herbs, fish, and, of course, fresh-cut flowers?

The term *artisanal* lately creeping into American restaurants and markets provides a clue. Handcrafted quality has
always been at the heart of French gastronomy and culture.
French women live by it. It encompasses handling as well as
production: eggs that are hours, not months, old, the yolks not
pale yellow, but orange and exploding with flavor. It means
white peaches picked early that morning, oozing with juices

and destined to live at peak intensity for but a day before slowly dying.

Faire son marché (to do one's food shopping) remains a vital French institution, here to stay despite the proliferation of the hypermarkets (now, mercifully, limited by law). It's a vital social occasion. We see our neighbors, compare notes, and, crucially, get to know the producers, the farmers who come to recognize you and whom you learn to trust. It's critically important, because in France one does not dare squeeze the merchandise; rather, the trusted purveyors pick among the produce for you according to when you plan to eat something, how, and with what. This discussion can go on a bit, and the next in line waits quite patiently, respecting the seriousness of her neighbor's business.

I was at a fruit stand in the Marché Saint-Germain, planning meals to follow Edward's imminent arrival from New York. Like a trained psychoanalyst, a wonderful vendor there probed me: *"C'est pour ce soir?"* ("Is it for tonight?") "Yes, the white peaches are, but the yellow ones are for tomorrow night." She looked and picked thoughtfully. I usually buy what I need for the same evening, but I knew I'd be at the office that day past market time, and I wanted to treat Edward to a melon (de Cavaillon), one of his favorite French fruits, for his first lunch in Paris on Saturday. As I turned to the melon bushel, she inquired, *"C'est pour quand?"* I told her and she went to work, weighing a few, considering the stems and scents; then, having narrowed it down to two, she finally said with a smile of certainty, *"Dans ce cas, c'est celui-ci."* She presented the one in her right hand, having calculated that the one in her left wouldn't be perfect until Sunday. Of course, one never stores fruit in the refrigerator, so I left her selection in the basket on the kitchen counter and forgot about it. On Saturday morning, excited with anticipation of Edward's arrival, I awoke to the most intoxicating fragrance permeating the apartment. The melon was crying, "Eat me," and when Edward showed up from the airport there was no way to keep it a surprise. He just said, "Wow," as he passed the kitchen.

If my market visits in New York are not quite as intense as those in Paris or Provence, they are still rich experiences in meeting and greeting produce and people; one can see and taste what's in season and learn how to prepare the season's local best with respect. Farmers universally love to share recipes, and Americans, being a curious and friendly bunch, are naturally unafraid to ask what to do with one foodstuff or another, be it skate, zucchini flowers, sorrel, or shallots. (Here you are at an advantage: sometimes French pride and fear of seeming ignorant restrain us, but one should never be discreet where food information is concerned.) Today, the thrill of outdoor markets is sweeping American cities from San Francisco to Santa Monica, Seattle, Chicago, Boston, and beyond. Chances are there is one near you. New York's nationally famous Union Square market is open four days a week. Naturally, the countryside is no less rich in opportunity, and far from dying out, the traditional farm stand is thriving from Long Island to Pennsylvania to California to Wisconsin.

Once you've bought fruit and vegetables in an open-air market, not to mention bread, eggs, chicken, and fish, it's hard to face the supermarket as anything more than a dry goods store. Obviously you must learn the market's rhythm. In France, we are spoiled by daily markets, but there are weekly ones as well. In Provence, for instance, the famous daily ones are in the cities of Nice, Aix, and Avignon, while among smaller towns a weekly one rotates. So if it's Tuesday, it's Vaison La Romaine; the next day will be Carpentras; after that, Ménerbes; Saint Rémy de Provence; Uzès; and so on. Keeping track of when and where to go isn't a bother, it's almost a sport we enjoy. The effort is repaid tenfold in the kitchen. The best cook in the world can't make good food from poor ingredients; and it takes some perverse genius to turn great ingredients into bad food. Good food in season responds best to the simplest preparation; you really can't go wrong when you start with quality.

The last twenty years have seen astonishing strides in American cooking, with a heartwarming new respect for *cuisine du terroir*, bringing the best of the earth onto the restaurant and home kitchen table. American apostles of this faith like Alice Waters were the first to get Americans thinking seriously about ingredients and markets, and there is nothing short of a revolution under way as more and more Americans are converted to the satisfactions of making it themselves.

One difference between America and France remains a bit of a paradox. America, the paragon of egalitarian values, somehow suffers from a gastronomic class system unknown in France. The right and the opportunity to enjoy the earth's seasonal best seems to be monopolized by an elite. Outside their ranks, the great majority of Americans are conditioned to demand and accept bland, processed, chemically treated, generally unnatural foods, which through packaging and marketing have been made to seem wholesome. I have no doubt that any people made to eat this way would in time grow fat.

Among the French, by contrast, a love of good, natural food is part of the universal patrimony. Not that the French don't pay more for quality. On average, they spend a much greater proportion of their income on food. But what seems like a luxury to Americans is a necessity to the French. Of course, not all luxury is within reach of everyone (the beluga appetizer is not a universal right), but the French do live by one principle that Americans sometimes forget, despite having coined it most eloquently: Garbage in, garbage out. The key to cooking, and therefore living well, is the best of ingredients.

Part of living like a French woman, then, will mean searching out and paying a bit more for quality, whether at the open-air market or at least a good grocery shop with market suppliers. This is now within the means of a great many more American women. French women live on budgets, too, but they also understand the value of quality over quantity.

Another issue, of course, is availability. And though the market in America has yet to become what it is in France, only a few are beyond the reach of quality on account of where people live. New markets and specialty food shops are cropping up everywhere across the country, especially with a surging demand for organically grown produce. One must take the trouble to find them. And thanks to the Internet, many quality foods not in driving (or better, walking) distance are but a mouse click away.

SEASONINGS

In any French market you'll find pots and pots of fresh herbs as well as rows and rows of dried herbs and spices. In cities and towns, grocery shops (*épiceries*) stock a decent range of spices. Though French food is hardly known for being spicy, French women could not do without seasonings. Artfully deployed, they are key to blissfully fooling ourselves, furnishing a world of flavors in recipes that might otherwise depend on fat for their tastiness. As you play with herbs and spices, keep in mind that the latter are by nature more pungent. Strive to become an adventurous seasoner, but learn your boldness *peu à peu.* A little turmeric goes far, and you can always add but never subtract.

The most common herbs in French cuisine are parsley, sweet basil, tarragon, thyme, lemon thyme, chervil, marjoram, oregano, rosemary—used in soups, meat, poultry, fish, vegetables, and salads—and sage, not typically used with fish and salads but great with meat and mushrooms. We chop them at the last second to enjoy maximum flavor. As for spices, we favor paprika, cayenne pepper, and increasingly curry and ginger, especially with poultry, meats, and vegetables. Of course, cinnamon and nutmeg are used mostly for desserts, but try, for example, a slight sprinkle of cinnamon on lamb, whether stewed or broiled, or add a dash of nutmeg to a chicken dish with cream or on veggies such as carrots, green beans, squash, or spinach. (The unexpected can be the greatest delight: the Alsace-born chef Jean-Georges Vongerichten caused a stir in New York when he flavored ice cream with ground pepper.)

Mustard is a most versatile condiment (invest in top quality; we French like Dijon, Pommery, and Meaux, each of which has a number of producers of varying quality). Adding some to a cream soup, a hamburger (a nice alternative to ketchup), cheese and egg dishes, sandwiches (instead of, or even more luxurious than, mayonnaise), salad dressing, a fish sauce, or any casserole lends an extra note and complexity. Fresh herbs like basil, mint, and rosemary are ideal for summer cooking, whereas in fall and winter dried herbs with spices will furnish the best accent for everything from lamb to fruit compote. Spices facilitate digestion of heavier foods and strengthen our immune system, which is challenged more severely in winter. So we use them more generously in the cold months. Both herbs and spices can also help you cut back on salt, which promotes water retention and temporary weight gain. (Even the fleeting impression of added pounds can be dispiriting when we mean to reduce!)

As you might expect, the quality of one's seasonings is *très important*. That's why the French use mills for both pepper and salt, grinding these staples at the last second to release fresh flavors the moment they are needed. Sea salt, much more intense than the standard iodized table variety, makes a world of taste difference. And did you know there are at least a dozen varieties of peppercorns? Nowadays you can grow your own herb garden with no trouble; savvy entrepreneurs have even created instant gardens—just add water and in a couple of weeks you have a tabletop farm. Learn by doing. In the city, I grow varieties of parsley, thyme, rosemary, mint, chives, and basil in my windowbox, from late spring till early fall, when I bring them inside to a sunny area. Basil doesn't respond well to life indoors, so at the end of the summer, I flatten and freeze individual leaves and also make a goodly supply of pesto. This I freeze in ice cube trays. I seal the individual frozen cubes in separate airtight packages that come in handy on cold December nights, when one provides ample instant sauce for one pasta serving.

Personally, I have a huge fondness for rosemary, with its pungent aroma and distinctive taste. I use it both fresh and dried as my preferred herb with lamb, Cornish hen, or any type of poultry. I was introduced to rosemary as a teenager vacationing in Provence. One of my relatives kept a pot in her bedroom because she believed the aroma was stimulating, cleansing, and comforting. Others also report this soothing effect on the nervous system. If you hold a sprig under your nose, you'll see what these Provençales are talking about.

Try a range of seasonings, and soon you'll learn which appeal to you most. Keep these in stock, but always remain open to new combinations of flavors. A few basic dishes can be varied dramatically by changing the way you season them (I have given examples of this in the next chapter). Just remember that here, too, "less is more." When you've learned to taste your food with care, you'll find yourself noticing the interplay of ingredients as never before. The more flavors you train yourself to register, the more complex your appreciation of taste will become. And a well-trained palate is quicker to reach contentment. Keeping your mind interested in what you're eating is fundamental to eating less and losing weight.

NUTS

We toss nuts in salads all the time and certainly sprinkle them on fish and even meats. We add them to pasta and crumble them over yogurt, cake, or ice cream. We extract from them fragrant oils that make a lovely alternative to the sacred *huile d'olive.*

Supremely nutritious, they can be a delicious and healthy accent in many a dish and presentation, making it considerably more substantial because of their concentration of good fats. But did you know nuts are seasonal?

If you have ever eaten fresh hazelnuts or almonds, you understand. It's perfectly reasonable when you remember they are fruits that grow on trees and bushes. I'm unapologetically nuts about nuts, and my favorite varieties are hazelnuts, walnuts, and almonds. Part of the attraction comes, I must admit, from having been spoiled as a child. Our garden had a few hazelnut (*noisette*) trees (which resemble large bushes) and a huge walnut (*noix*) tree, and there were also rows of hazelnut trees behind my grandmother's home in Alsace. There's nothing like cracking a freshly fallen nut; the thin, brown envelope is so supple, it surrenders the sweet white meat without a fight. The smell and taste are indescribable, as far from a bag of airplane nuts as a fine *saucisson* is from a Slim-Jim.

Years later, visiting friends in Greece, I would experience fresh almonds (even more delicate and with a most sensual touch of sweetness). When I returned to France, I put up a poster of Bonnard's *L'Amandier en Fleurs* in my room to remind me of that experience. At home in the fall, we always had a bowl of fresh nuts, and after the Sunday meal we would pass it around just before coffee. We kids loved to crack them open. (Storing them uncracked preserves flavor and helps you enjoy fewer, making you work for the calories.) *Mamie* would pack handfuls in tiny brown bags to be eaten during the ten a.m. recess in the schoolyard. Our *nounou* (nanny), Yvette, a sweet young lady who was practically adopted by our family, claimed this and other good foods were the secret to our excellent grades.

A small handful of unsalted raw nuts is still one of my favorite snacks, sometimes part of lunch, and an emergency travel food (the *en-cas,* often including a few pieces of dried fruit, especially apricots, that I keep in my pocketbook for the departure lounge). Nuts are rich in beneficial monounsaturated fat as well as good sources of vitamin E, folate, potassium, magnesium, zinc, and other minerals essential to health. Many people think of nuts as a high-calorie, high-fat food, which is true, so practice moderation: those six or eight nuts (about one ounce) are the equivalent of, say, two ounces of chicken but are far richer in vital nutrients. Have a small handful and reap the healthful benefits. Savor them one by one.

Most of what we find in shops is typically months old and sometimes rancid. On airplanes or in lounges, the offerings are hardly any better, often heavy on the salt to cover staleness. Securing nuts at their prime can be an adventure in quality. After I moved to New York, I still regularly visited my parents in France, and my mother remained my key supplier. I always had a big bag of hazelnuts to take back home to New York. One year, I was preparing the Thanksgiving meal and had a wonderful recipe for pumpkin pie requiring a base of pecans. I didn't have any and decided to substitute my fresh hazelnuts. To this day, Edward, who loves pumpkin pie, claims this is the best he's ever had (another lesson in the pleasures of serendipity). Now, I order my hazelnuts from Oregon right after harvest and find them closest to what I grew up eating. If you can't get freshly picked, at least make sure they are not stale. Health food stores tend to have the best retail turnover. You should store them in an airtight jar away from the light (and please, not in the refrigerator).

PUMPKIN PIE WITH HAZELNUTS

Serves 10

1. Put the flour, pinch of salt, and sugar in the bowl of a food processor and pulse to combine.

2. Cut the chilled butter into small pieces and add to the bowl. Also add the water and process for 15 seconds. If the dough is too dry, add more water by droplets. The dough should just hold together. Do not knead.

3. Wrap the dough in waxed paper and refrigerate at least 4 hours or overnight.

4. Preheat the oven to 400 degrees. Roll out the pastry and fit it into a 9-inch pie plate, 2 inches deep. Prick the pastry with a fork all over the bottom. Line the pie plate with aluminum foil. Add pie weights or dried beans to weigh down the dough, and bake for 10 minutes in the preheated oven. Remove from the oven and discard foil and beans.

5. Increase the oven temperature to 450 degrees. Prepare the filling by combining hazelnuts, 1/4 cup granulated brown sugar, and butter. Work into a paste and spread with the back of a fork or a rubber spatula into the partially cooked pastry shell. Bake for 10 minutes.

INGREDIENTS

PIECRUST:

2/3 cup unsifted flour

Pinch of salt

1 tablespoon sugar

6 tablespoons chilled butter

1½ tablespoons ice cold water

FILLING:

1/3 cup ground hazelnuts

1/4 cup granulated brown sugar

2 tablespoons softened butter

2 eggs, plus 1 egg yolk

1 cup unsweetened canned pumpkin purée (organic, natural preferred)

1 tablespoon flour

2/3 cup granulated brown sugar

1/4 teaspoon cinnamon

1/4 teaspoon ground cloves

1/2 teaspoon salt

1 cup heavy cream

6. Mix together the eggs, egg yolk, pumpkin purée, flour, 2/3 cup granulated brown sugar, spices, salt, and heavy cream. Pour into the pastry shell. Turn the oven temperature down to 325 degrees and bake the pie for 45 minutes.

7. Serve at room temperature or cold. Optional: Serve with unsweetened whipped cream (1 cup for the entire pie) on the side.

N.B. THE PIE WILL KEEP A FEW DAYS IN THE REFRIGERATOR. ALWAYS TAKE OUT 15 MINUTES BEFORE SERVING.

. . . .

OTHER FRUITS

Growing up French means eating lots of fruit—in season, that is. We certainly did in my family. Our garden had rows and rows of strawberries, one huge cherry tree covered with the big, juicy, two-color variety, and a small one bearing sour cherries; raspberry and blackberry bushes grew like weeds along the stone walls and near the walnut and hazelnut trees. And in various parcels there were jumbles of rhubarb, onions, leeks, tomatoes, and carrots with other fruit bushes of *groseilles* (red currants) and larger varieties (like *maquereaux*) destined mostly for jellies and jams.

Every year before the end of school, I would be allowed to have a party around the big cherry tree. With our gardener on hand as lifeguard, my friends and I would take turns climbing. I had an advantage, being the most practiced, but a few brave others would join me on the high limbs to pick cherries we would throw down to the less bold. By the end, all our mouths were stained shades of red and purple. The part I sometimes repress is that year after year there was always one who would overdo it, paying dearly afterward with *un petit mal d'estomac.* Moderation is best learned early.

Strawberry season meant a strawberry cure. They were, then as now, my favorite fruit, and for about six weeks we would have them almost every day for dessert, picking them literally minutes before eating them. My father was obsessive with his crops, and in springtime we'd all pitch in laying some straw on the ground between the bunches so that when the green berries had bloomed and soaked in enough sun to ripen, they would rest on the straw, not the soil, allowing us to eat them unwashed. (It was a primal pleasure that at first shocked my American husband with his heightened sense of hygiene; but he got used to it and never had a stomachache.)

Six weeks of even one's favorite might have seemed monotonous were it not for the great range of variations: Monday was the day when Mother had the least time to be fancy; so at lunch we would have them plain, picking from a big bowl in the middle of the table. Most other days, we would have *fraises à la crème,* something one does not get in restaurants. My mother would gently mash the ripe strawberries with a fork, allowing the scarlet juices to flow; after adding a little sugar, she would let the mixture rest at room temperature until lunchtime. By then, the aroma was calling to us irresistibly, and mixing in just a dab of crème fraîche was enough to obtain a luscious light pink soup (the very thought makes my mouth water). If we served it on the tiny white dessert plates with the gold border (a trick for making small portions look larger), it was possible to have seconds and feel richly satisfied.

Sundays were pie days, and my mother would make a *tarte aux fraises.* After selecting a basket of perfect specimens, all of similar size, she would bake a delicious *pâte brisée* or *pâte sablée,* let it cool, and align the raw strawberry tips to point upward. With a strawberry coulis to glaze them and *crème chantilly* (whipped cream) on the side, this was prettier than anything you could see in the fanciest pastry shop and utterly delicious, with far fewer calories.

In wintertime, she'd follow the same recipe with the sour cherries, and we absolutely loved the tartness of the pie. What we loved less was the picking, pitting, and preserving (in sterilized glass jars) that we all had to assist in on summer Sunday evenings, although Mother was always quick to remind us how we would love the cherry pies in winter when there was not much fresh fruit around. (Fruit is one of those rare foods whose enjoyment out of season is an art in itself, and few know their preserves as French women do.) *Mamie* also had a few sour cherry variations: raw (only the women in the family loved them that way), in pies, or best of all, for those fancy Sunday lunches, when she would make Dad's favorite dessert, *baba au rhum.* Instead of soaking the cake with a lot of rum, she would use the juice from the preserved cherries, adding just a dash of rum to moisten the *baba.* Before serving, she would pour the cherries from the vacuum-sealed glass jar into the hole of the large baked *baba,* then top it with whipped cream. This was a rare treat, not usually made at home and always requested by our guests, who were the only ones allowed a second serving.

Raspberries and mulberries were mostly eaten plain in season, but we had so many that Mother would always freeze some (a preserving method that fails miserably with strawberries, adding to their mystique, but works well with most other berries). For one of our favorite winter desserts, usually enjoyed on Sundays, Mother would make a vanilla pudding topped with the berries, their juices flowing down the shimmering sides—not only lovely to behold but uniquely delicious, with the thick but subtle flavor of the pudding, just slightly sweetened, contrasting with the soft mushiness of the defrosted berries and the perfumed coulis.

As for other berries, in Alsace they abounded in nature beyond our garden wall. With a big wooden stick she used as a cane for forest walks, my grandmother would lead the family on expeditions. In the woods behind her house was the most incredible field of *myrtille* (wild blueberry) bushes, her secret garden. We were each charged with filling a little container, but I would fall behind trying to fill my mouth as well. My grandmother needed a lot of *myrtilles* to make a pie, as these tiny fruits have nothing to do with the marble-size berries we find in the United States. They are also noticeably tastier, at once sweet and sour, but also somewhat spicy. Sometimes by the end my father would have to help me meet my quota, sharing some of his pickings. I remember trying to describe *myrtilles* to Edward. He couldn't quite get it until he had an epiphany a few years later at l'Auberge de l'Îll, a gastronomic shrine in Alsace, where for dessert they served the first *tarte aux myrtilles* of the season. I wish I had a picture of his face at that moment.

In most of the world, summer means peaches and melons followed by pears and, into the fall, apples. In France, we seem to have an obsession for following the varieties of plums that appear from late summer into the fall. Indeed, we consume about 40 million pounds per year. Back home, the season would start at the very end of summer with *la mirabelle,* a variety unique to eastern France. It's a small, round, juicy, sweet little yellow thing the size of a cherry tomato, with a subtle perfume close to vanilla and honey. We use it in tarts, sauces (like applesauce), preserves, sorbets, and *alcools blancs,* the clear fiery distilled spirits my grandfather would drink after a big meal to facilitate digestion. We are so serious about these plums that there is such a thing as *la fête de la Mirabelle:* a queen is chosen and paraded through town, followed by trucks loaded with the plums. There are organized tastings covering every manner of preparation. And competitions. My mother's was pretty good, but I must say that *Tante* Berthe's was the best, which is why she would never reveal the recipe. I did manage, as a teenager, to catch her in the act of preparation, but she made me promise to keep this one *en famille,* so I don't include it here.

A more common variety in France is *la quetsche,* the elongated, juicy plum with a violet color and a firm flesh. In the fall, I make *clafoutis* and tarts with them. Often labeled as Italian plums in the United States, they freeze well for winter treats. I frequently use the ones squirreled away in the freezer as an accompaniment to *panna cotta,* the Italian custard. The *panna cotta* itself takes about five minutes (plus four hours in the fridge to set), and another five are needed to cook the defrosted plums in a bit of butter and sprinkle them with the tiniest mixture of sugar and cinnamon to complement the custard's flavor and texture.

Finally, there is the variety I eat all year long as part of my personal wellness program. Called *la prune d'Ente,* it is a violet plum used in southwestern France to make the famous *pruneaux d'Agen,* or Agen prunes. Edward used to make fun of me because I still eat two prunes at breakfast a few times a week—it seems to him too unglamorous to be French. But prunes are packed with vitamins and, of course, high in fiber, as the old jokes tell us, a mild laxative loaded with potassium, calcium, and magnesium. French women consider prunes the perfect detox food; they purify the body and help maintain a good balance in trace elements, so children should be taught to like them. They are good for everyone, not just old folks.

No discussion of French fruit preferences could exclude the lemon. If you've ever taken a *boisson* with a French woman on a sunny café terrace, you know she'll often go for a *citron pressé* before (or instead of) an espresso or mineral water. It's basically the juice of a lemon to which one adds cold or warm water (no sugar, please). You can even have it with breakfast (half a lemon will do). We also enjoy an idea borrowed from Italy, the *canarino:* the zest of a fresh lemon steeped as tea. Acquiring the taste for lemon is an excellent stabilization habit.

Fruit consumption is one of the most telling differences between French and American eating patterns. Too many American women eat too little, if any, and who can blame them, considering their reliance on the supermarket, with its tasteless offerings, waxed and rushed unripe to the shelves? Fruit is a staple of French life, and you must make it a staple of yours. And there is no excuse, as it is the one food easily enjoyed without preparation. You simply have to know what is available and when and what can be preserved for the off-season. Making your way once a week to where the good stuff is sold is one of the easiest ways to increase quality. If you can make it to market, you can have one of eating's greatest pleasures at your disposal! If not, oranges and grapefruits shipped fresh from Florida from late November into February are a real treat and an antidote to the paucity of local fruits during winter.

PLUM *CLAFOUTIS* WITHOUT DOUGH

Serves 4

The classic clafoutis (fruit tart) is naturally richer with batter. But as I learned from Dr. Miracle, the flourless version, properly seasoned, can give you the impression of indulgence with far fewer calories. A tiny scoop of ice cream is a good countermeasure, too. I often prepare this dessert at home when I want to compensate for the richness of an earlier course and to inject some fruit nutrients and fiber into the meal. It also provides a trick for handling not quite ripe plums—a little cooking and a dash of sugar make all the difference. The same recipe works with cherries, apples, pears, or figs.

INGREDIENTS

12 plums
1 tablespoon lemon juice
1 tablespoon sugar
¼ teaspoon cinnamon
1 teaspoon butter

1. Wash the plums and quarter them. Pour the lemon juice over and marinate for 10 minutes.

2. Mix the sugar with the cinnamon. Warm the butter in a nonstick frying pan and add the plums. Sprinkle with the sugar-cinnamon mixture.

3. Cook over low flame till just tender but not mushy (a bit al dente is best). Serve at room temperature with or without ice cream.

. . . .

BLUEBERRY BABY SMOOTHIE
Serves 4

This versatile, very healthy drink, especially rich in antioxidants, can be the better part of your lunch, snack, or even breakfast (though I prefer a more robust and balanced start to the day), as well as a dessert partner accompanying a cookie or warm dessert muffin. I discovered it as a child, again visiting my grandmother in Alsace, where we picked many more wild blueberries in the forests than we could possibly eat in season. Blueberries freeze extremely well. Today, I buy quarts and quarts of blueberries at the height of their season from the farmers' market for immediate freezing. Voilà, blueberries year-round. The following drink, an old-fashioned version of the modern smoothie (rien de nouveau sous le soleil—nothing new under the sun), includes a little kicker.

1. Take the blueberries out of the freezer 30 minutes before using.

2. Mix the blueberries in a blender with the lemon juice, honey, and milk. Add a sprinkle of cardamom before serving.

INGREDIENTS

12 ounces frozen blueberries

2 tablespoons lemon juice

2 tablespoons honey

2 1/4 cups 2 percent milk

Pinch of ground cardamom

The quintessential ingredient in Provençal cuisine is also known as *la pomme d'amour*—the apple of love. Tomatoes, as every schoolchild knows, are fruit. And unless cooked, I recommend they be eaten in season. There is nothing I long for more in winter than a real tomato when none are to be had. But it only makes the fruit of summer all the more precious. Don't be tempted by a pretty face alone. Wait for the season.

I weather the off-season with select cherry tomatoes (good ones available year-round) and limit my tomato cure to a few summer months, finding beefy New Jersey heirlooms and other excellent local varieties at the Union Square market, but good tomatoes can be found across America throughout the summer. Plus, they are rich in vitamins A and C and a good source of folate, potassium, and other healthful nutrients.

Remember, except for the uncommon yellow variety (a nice visual variation in any tomato recipe), ripe tomatoes are brilliant red. But good color alone is not sufficient proof. If they don't smell ripe (or at all), then they aren't. Don't put them in the refrigerator, ever, if you want to experience their full and natural flavors. Leave them on your counter and wash them just before you use them. In the winter, tomato purée lends a sweet thickness to many a sauce.

TOMATO SALAD WITH GOAT CHEESE

Serves 4

Although you can find tomatoes year-round in France, too, they just aren't the same as they are in season, which runs June through September. In summer, my family used to eat tomatoes at least twice a week, but typically three or four times, in different raw preparations for full flavor. In this recipe, a bit of cheese makes for a heartier dish, which means the meat or fish portion later in the meal can be smaller or eliminated. We almost always had some fresh goat cheese from a local farm, but you can add mozzarella as in Italy or feta as they do in Greece.

1. Cover each plate with a layer of mesclun or mixed greens. Place sliced tomatoes on top. Salt generously.

2. Mix the dressing ingredients into an emulsion.

3. Crumble the goat cheese onto the tomato slices.

4. Season with salt and pepper to taste. Pour the dressing on top. Add the chopped parsley. Serve with a slice of country bread.

INGREDIENTS

Mesclun or any mixed salad greens, about 1 cup per person

4 large tomatoes, washed and sliced

SALAD DRESSING:

2 tablespoons minced shallots

1 teaspoon mustard

2 tablespoons vinegar

6 tablespoons olive oil

8 ounces fresh goat cheese

Salt and freshly ground pepper

4 tablespoons parsley (or basil)—chopped at the last minute!

No question about it, the French eat a lot more mushrooms, in total quantity and variety, than Americans. There's genuine excitement each fall as more and more fresh mushrooms are brought to markets. Fine-restaurant menus highlight mushroom preparations, and the all-mushroom tasting menu is often featured as a treat.

In agrarian and densely forested France, mushrooming was once a simple seasonal chore. Today, it's an outdoor adventure sport and popular hobby. One of the priceless charms of wild mushroom picking is the aromas of the fields and the *sous-bois* (forest floor). When I was a kid, we'd leave right after breakfast, the morning dew still hanging on every leaf. The smell of wet dead leaves was mysterious and captivating (to this day, I can summon it up only in tasting some red wines and old Champagnes or smelling a particular type of tobacco). When we saw mushrooms we didn't know for sure to be edible, we brought them to my grandmother, who was an expert; others sought out the pharmacist. (Admittedly, only the least and the most experienced mushroom pickers ever seem to die of poisoning; the rest of us are not so bold.)

It's not difficult to find mushrooms year-round in America. I speak of the ones grown in moist industrial basements somewhere. You know them: white and perfect looking, with round half-moon button tops. There are worse things you could eat than these clones, but ugly mushrooms are far tastier, and the freshly picked ones are indescribably good. Fine mushrooms are available in gourmet shops (where some can be poisonously expensive) and in outdoor markets (where they are not cheap, either). But with mushrooms you should bite the bullet of cost. Avoid the supermarket, and consider this something to splurge on when you can.

Grandmère was also expert in mushroom handling, and she taught my mother how to dry them and also to preserve them via sterilization. A good dried mushroom is better than a poor fresh one. But nothing beats a fine fresh one, and among fresh, the wild ones reign supreme. Chanterelles, also called girolles (yellow orange), and *trompettes de la mort* (black) were accompaniments to many dishes through the spring, particularly veal, rabbit, and game. Our favorite recipe was the simplest, *fricassée de champignons sauvages*. The mushrooms are cleaned without water, with only a clean, dry towel and paring knife. A bit of oil and butter is put in the frying pan, and when it's sizzling hot, the mushrooms are sautéed with some very finely sliced shallots, lemon juice, parsley, and salt and pepper. That appetizer with a glass of Champagne is, to my mind and palate, one of the greatest food-and-wine pairings. Many years later, I rediscovered that dish at Les Crayères, the top restaurant in Reims, and it reconfirmed my grandmother's unfailing intuition with wine and food. An Italian friend later shared a recipe for mushroom flan with mascarpone cheese and Parmesan that is equally excellent with Champagne.

Mushrooms have been enjoyed for thousands of years; the ancient Chinese loved them and noted their probiotic benefits. Although we've greatly increased the farmed varieties, we still don't quite understand the mystery of perfect mushroom growth. So if you're near some meadow or forest where you can pick them (with a reliable judge of safety), consider yourself blessed. For all their satisfying taste and texture, mushrooms contain almost no fat, sugar, or salt but are a good source of dietary fiber and are richer in proteins than most other fresh vegetables. They are filled with vitamins and minerals, especially B vitamins, but these are lost when they are cooked in boiling water, so consider eating them raw (with a light oil dressing)—which seems all but inconceivable with the supermarket kind. We should all consume mushrooms regularly: raw or cooked, not to mention stuffed.

SALMON AND OTHER THINGS THAT SWIM

If you were born not too long ago and live in a city, you probably think that virtually all varieties of fish are available year-round, especially salmon. You see it everywhere, now more than ever since it has been touted as the cure for everything from heart disease to wrinkles. We've all heard that eating salmon, with its extraordinary concentration of good fats, lowers blood pressure, thins blood, dilates blood vessels, regulates the heartbeat, and fights cancer, among many other benefits. But remember those nature films of the salmon's heroic swim upstream to spawn in the spring, most dying in the attempt? Real salmon is seasonal food.

To meet the skyrocketing year-round demand, the bulk of salmon today comes from huge farms that create awful environmental pressures as well as salmon relatively poor in the nutrients that caused the fish to be declared a wonder food. I've been salmon fishing in Alaska and eaten my catch for lunch. There's no comparison between the color and taste of what is passing for salmon and wild native salmon, which in most parts of the country is now about twice as expensive.

This is just supply and demand: there isn't enough good salmon to go around. But more is unquestionably less where salmon is concerned. Although it loses some taste and texture, you are better off buying frozen wild salmon (Alaskan variety or, in any case, Pacific, available most abundantly in late spring in the Northern Hemisphere but in lesser quantities elsewhere during the year, especially as the wild variety swim the oceans far and wide) than buying farmed.

There's nary a restaurant in France without salmon in some form; in pre-farm days it came from Norway or Scotland (still the European gourmet's choice). The most common of all presentations is *saumon fumé* (smoked salmon), perfect as an appetizer at dinner parties or cocktails because there is no preparation. Smoked salmon on toast with a glass of Champagne is a classic (the oiliness and saltiness of salmon work marvels with the acidity of Champagne). Salmon is so versatile, it lends itself to every taste: pair a few ounces of the good stuff, smoked, raw, or cooked (served warm or cold), with potatoes, rice, leeks, fennel—any of your favorite vegetables. Salmon is flattered by dill, basil, cumin, capers, lemon, and many other accents. Try salmon with sorrel sauce, a simple but elegant dish to make at home. But for simplicity, nothing beats *Saumon à l'Unilatéral,* which I always serve in a pinch because it takes exactly six minutes to prepare.

My uncle Charles owned a spa hotel, and in the early days of nouvelle cuisine he taught me the simple, foolproof ways of eating light but tasty. He used to prepare this dish for his more ambivalent guests. They were paying for a "cure" but had an inclination to indulge because of a vacation mind-set.

It's a useful lesson: no one wants to pay for deprivation. This incredibly simple and healthy dish was a good solution, he felt, for those who insisted on ending meals with *l'omelette norvégienne,* just about the richest ice cream dessert in all of France.

SAUMON À L'UNILATÉRAL
(COOKED ON ONE SIDE ONLY)
Serves 4

1. Heat a nonstick frying pan. Place the salmon in the pan, skin-side down, pour the lemon juice over the salmon, add the salt, and cook for about 6 minutes over medium heat until the skin is crispy. (Cut a slice to determine the degree of cooking you desire, such as medium-rare—pink at the center—which preserves most of the natural taste.)

2. Serve immediately. Season, if you like, with a dash of extra-virgin olive oil and a sprig of fresh thyme.

INGREDIENTS

4 pieces of wild salmon, about 4 ounces each

1 tablespoon fresh lemon juice

½ teaspoon coarse salt

. . . .

When there isn't salmon, there is something else. Each weekend I visit the fish stall at the Union Square market and buy skate or tuna that is only hours out of the water. Top New York chefs come here or go directly to the wholesale fish market. Admittedly, the fish market—and every port city has one—is not a stroll in the botanical gardens. Few nonprofessionals will have the time or inclination, but try it once to see the difference. For one thing, fresh fish does not smell fishy. Its flesh does not look shellacked. If you can tell quality, it's possible to find it at a good grocery store. It saves time: good fish is the simplest thing in the world to cook.

I love sea scallops, those sweet, nutty, fleshy medallions that have a normal season from perhaps late October or early November through March. That's the only time most restaurants in Brittany, France's seafood mecca, will serve them. Scallops are especially popular at year's end, as I was reminded at my favorite Paris bistro, Benoît, one November. It's one of those places where everything's *comme il faut,* but nevertheless I asked the seasoned waiter, "What's good today?"

"Madame," he replied, as though pained for me, "the scallops, of course!" He was right.

Oysters are another singular eating experience. Not nearly as expensive as, say, caviar, but somehow they speak of the utmost sophistication in the twenty-first century (in the nineteenth, they were inexpensive, common, and a bit proletarian). And what could be easier to serve? It was Escoffier, the legendary Parisian chef, who at the turn of the twentieth century introduced the practice of serving them over a bed of crushed ice with their half shells as little bowls for the delicious salty juices. A quick squeeze of lemon and a few twists of pepper wonderfully complement the natural flavor. And though oysters are an acquired taste, once you try them, you might find yourself hooked on the sensation of that tender grayish glob of seagoing goodness sliding down your throat. Not for nothing do hedonists pair oyster eating with seduction. And some will add that the true sensual delight is enhanced by watching another savor them with you.

My husband likes to tell a story of our first trip to discover Brittany, early in our marriage. For him that meant the landscape, the sea, the similarities with England, the architecture, the history. I was interested in those things, too, but frankly I was more eager to experience Brittany's mussels, oysters, crêpes, and wondrous variety of cookies. We headed first to a beautiful little auberge near the sea to visit the oyster beds. A little shack nearby served them by the dozen, and though it was early for lunch, we had to have some. We sat there, alone, ordered, and the next thing I can remember is Edward laughing out loud. Gazing into the platter set before us, I had totally lost awareness of being there with someone else, entranced by the smell of seawater and of its precious fruit. As I concentrated on swallowing these firm little morsels, Edward said he had never seen anyone "experience" oysters that way. And it was only our second dozen.

The next day, I showed him how we eat mussels: no fork necessary, just use your first two half-empty shells and scoop out the meat of each mussel. With a glass or two of Muscadet, we had fabulous lunches, low in calories, high in minerals and vitamins. Oysters, too, can be the main element of a surprisingly balanced meal, containing protein, carbohydrates, and just a little fat (to say nothing of the wealth of vitamins and minerals). I'm always amazed that half a dozen oysters are only sixty or seventy calories. Like a great love, they give a lot back, always new, never boring. When we are in Paris, places like Le Dôme that serve them brilliantly have become our cafeteria, and now, more than ever, there are wondrous varieties of oysters to be found in raw bars across America. Thanks to good cultivation practices filling steady but not exploding demand, the season is rather long: virtually year-round, but at its peak in the fall and winter. (The rule about the months ending with "r" comes from the days before refrigeration. Nevertheless, be careful during the summer months.) We French count oysters as one of our year-end rituals. Visit a French market at Christmas and especially on New Year's Eve and you'll see crate after crate awaiting indulgent mouths across the country.

PUTTING IT ALL TOGETHER

Seasonal menu planning becomes easy once you learn what's best when and pair it with your favorite flavors. Following are some examples of menus that are particularly good for stabilization. When you're beyond that, you can substitute richer elements—for instance, *clafoutis* made *with* dough.

· Spring *Menu du Jour* ·

Breakfast

Yogurt
Cereal with strawberries
Slice of whole-wheat or multigrain bread
Coffee or tea

Lunch

Asparagus Flan (page 104)
Green salad
Cherry *clafoutis* without dough (see recipe for Plum *Clafoutis,*
    page 90)
Noncaloric beverage

Dinner

Pea soup
Grilled Spring Lamb Chops (page 105)
Cauliflower Gratin (page 106)
Rhubarb compote
Glass of red wine

ASPARAGUS FLAN

Serves 4

INGREDIENTS

16 asparagus stalks

4 ounces bacon, coarsely chopped

8 eggs

2 cups milk

1 cup heavy cream

8 sprigs of fresh chervil, minced

Salt and freshly ground pepper

1. Cut off the tough ends of the asparagus stalks (about 2 inches). Peel the asparagus. Boil the asparagus in salted water for 5 minutes. Drain and let cool. Chop each stalk into 2- or 3-inch pieces.

2. Sauté the bacon in a nonstick frying pan till crisp. Drain on a paper towel.

3. Combine the eggs, milk, cream, and half of the chervil. Season with salt and pepper. Preheat the oven to 350 degrees. Pour the egg mixture in a 9-inch pie plate, 2 inches deep. Sprinkle in the asparagus and bacon. Bake for 15 to 20 minutes, till the custard is set but not dried out. Serve immediately, decorated with the rest of the chervil.

N.B. IF YOU DON'T WANT TO USE BACON, YOU CAN REPLACE IT WITH CRABMEAT, FRESH OR CANNED.

PARSLEY OR CHIVES CAN BE USED AS ALTERNATIVES TO CHERVIL.

. . . .

GRILLED SPRING LAMB CHOPS

Serves 4

1. Lay the chops in a baking dish.

2. Combine the olive oil, mustard, shallots, and mint in the bowl of a food processor and pulse till a medium-textured paste is formed. Spread the minty paste on each side of the chops, season them with salt and pepper, and let marinate at room temperature for 30 minutes.

3. Broil or grill the chops 3 minutes on each side for medium-rare meat. Serve immediately.

INGREDIENTS

8 spring lamb chops

4 tablespoons olive oil

1 tablespoon Dijon mustard

4 medium shallots

1 cup fresh mint

Salt and freshly ground pepper

CAULIFLOWER GRATIN

Serves 4

1 medium-size head of cauliflower

2 cups milk

½ teaspoon salt

1 egg

½ cup grated cheese (Gruyère, Swiss, Jarlsberg, Comté, Parmesan, or Pecorino, or a mix of 2)

1 tablespoon butter

Salt and freshly ground pepper

1. Trim the cauliflower, separate the flowerets, and cook in the milk and the ½ teaspoon of salt until tender (10 to 15 minutes). Drain, reserving ⅓ cup of the milk.

2. Arrange the cooked flowerets in a lightly buttered baking dish. Beat together the egg and reserved milk. Add the cheese and spread over the flowerets. Add salt and pepper. Dot with the butter.

3. Broil the gratin until browned and bubbly. Serve hot.

• Summer *Menu du Jour* •

Breakfast

Sliver of cheese
½ cup muesli with blueberries
Coffee or tea

Lunch

Bacon, lettuce, and tomato sandwich
Cup of raspberries
Noncaloric beverage

Dinner

Grilled Chicken with Rosemary (page 108)
Fennel gratin
Arugula salad
Grilled Peaches with Lemon Thyme (page 109)
Glass of white or red wine

GRILLED CHICKEN WITH ROSEMARY

Serves 4

INGREDIENTS

4 chicken breasts with skin
and bones

Juice of 1 lemon

4 tablespoons olive oil

4 garlic cloves, finely
minced

Fresh rosemary sprigs

Salt and freshly ground
pepper

1. Place the chicken breasts in a baking dish skin-side up. Mix together the lemon juice, olive oil, garlic, and rosemary sprigs and pour over chicken. Season with salt and pepper. (You can also do this in 5 minutes in the morning.) Cover with plastic wrap and marinate at least 2 hours in refrigerator.

2. Bring the chicken to room temperature before grilling, skin-side up, for 15 minutes and then skin-side down for 20 minutes.

GRILLED PEACHES WITH LEMON THYME

Serves 4

Peaches are such a delicate fruit, it's difficult—even in season—to find specimens perfect for eating raw. For this dessert, it does not matter; even hard ones will do, as the cooking will tenderize and release juices and flavors.

1. Rinse the peaches, pat dry, cut in half, and remove the pits. Place the peach halves in a baking dish. Mix together the olive oil, honey, and vanilla extract and pour over the peaches. Sprinkle with the lemon thyme. Marinate for 20 minutes, turning over once and basting.

2. Broil or grill the marinated peaches on the barbecue for 2 to 3 minutes on each side, or until the peaches are tender but not soft. Serve immediately, alone or with a scoop of vanilla ice cream.

INGREDIENTS

4 peaches

2 tablespoons olive oil

1 teaspoon honey

¼ teaspoon pure vanilla extract

4 sprigs lemon thyme, coarsely chopped

• Fall *Menu du Jour* •

Breakfast

Half grapefruit
Egg Omelet with Mixed Herbs and Ricotta Cheese (page 111)
Slice of bread (whole-wheat, multigrain, sourdough)
Coffee or tea

Lunch

Lentil Soup (page 127)
Caesar salad
Plums
Noncaloric beverage

Dinner

Halibut *en Papillote* (page 112)
Mushroom timbale
Cooked Pears with Cinnamon (page 114)
Glass of Champagne or white wine

EGG OMELET WITH MIXED HERBS AND RICOTTA CHEESE

Serves 4

I find this a wonderful weekend breakfast, especially when you have guests. It's a filling main dish preceded by some fruit and bread, and it can be prepared just before you sit down and served with a variety of breads (whole-wheat, seven-grain, and sourdough make for a good combination and accompaniment to the herbs and the sweet-sour flavors).

1. Wash and chop all the herbs and mix with the shallot, pimento, and cayenne pepper. Heat the olive oil in a nonstick frying pan. Add the herb mixture and cook for 1 minute, stirring constantly. Remove from the pan and reserve.

2. Beat together the eggs and water. Add the seasoning mixture, salt, and pepper. Melt the butter in the pan and add the egg-herb mixture. Stir till omelet starts setting, then add the cheese. Cook for 3 to 4 minutes and serve immediately or when lukewarm.

INGREDIENTS

2 tablespoons each of fresh parsley, chives, chervil, and coriander

1 shallot, minced

1 teaspoon pimento

Sprinkle of cayenne pepper

1 tablespoon olive oil

10 eggs

2 tablespoons water

Salt and freshly ground pepper

1 tablespoon butter

4 tablespoons ricotta or mascarpone cheese

HALIBUT *EN PAPILLOTE*

Serves 4

This is another simple dish that can be prepared in advance and put in the oven as your guests enjoy the appetizer. I believe in the principle of eating fish once or twice a week. But I notice lots of unpracticed cooks are intimidated by the notion of preparing fish, especially whole, so I'm always on the lookout for quick and easy preparations. You can substitute flounder, sole, monkfish, salmon, cod, bass, or swordfish for the halibut in this recipe. The cooking time will be shorter with lighter fish, such as sole, and longer with meatier fish, such as swordfish.

INGREDIENTS

2 teaspoons olive oil

4 fillets of halibut, about 4 ounces each

½ cup Champagne (Veuve Clicquot Yellow Label Brut recommended)

8 sprigs fresh thyme

8 thin lemon slices

8 sprigs parsley

2 teaspoons fennel seeds

Salt and freshly ground pepper

1. Cut 8 pieces of parchment paper (or aluminum foil) into squares large enough to cover each fish fillet and leave a 2-inch border all around. Lightly brush 4 squares of the paper with olive oil. Preheat the oven to 350 degrees.

2. Put each halibut fillet in the center of an oiled square and drizzle with Champagne. Add 2 sprigs of thyme, 2 lemon slices, 2 parsley sprigs, and ½ teaspoon fennel seeds to each piece of fish. Season with salt and pepper.

3. Place the remaining parchment squares on top of the fillets and fold up the edges to form packets. Simply double folding each of the four sides is enough to seal each

packet. Put the *papillotes* on a baking sheet and bake in the pre-heated oven for 10 to 15 minutes.

4. Serve by setting each *papillote* on a plate. Let your guests open their packets and spoon the juices over the fish. Voilà—drama as well as flavor!

N.B. YOU CAN USE DRY WHITE WINE OR VERMOUTH INSTEAD OF CHAMPAGNE.

COOKED PEARS WITH CINNAMON

Serves 4

INGREDIENTS

4 Bosc pears

Juice of 1 lemon

1 tablespoon sugar mixed
with ¼ teaspoon cinnamon

2 tablespoons water (or 2
tablespoons pear brandy or
2 tablespoons Muscat
Beaumes de Venise)

1. Peel, quarter, and thinly slice each pear, one at a time, placing the slices at the bottom of a 6-inch saucepan. After the slices of each pear are layered, sprinkle some lemon juice and sugar-cinnamon mixture over the slices. When you reach the fourth pear, add the water and then end with the remaining lemon juice and sugar-cinnamon mixture.

2. Cook over medium heat till boiling, and then cover and continue over a low flame until the pears are tender but not soft. Serve the pears lukewarm. (I often make this dessert when we are alone and refrigerate the other 2 servings, which 2 days later I remove from the refrigerator while I make dinner and serve at room temperature with biscotti or a teaspoon of mascarpone cheese.)

· ·

• Winter *Menu du Jour* •

Breakfast

Sliver of prosciutto
Grandma Louise's Oatmeal with Grated Apple (see page 116)
English muffin half
Coffee or tea

Lunch

Veal Parmesan
Squash
Kiwi
Noncaloric beverage

Dinner

Soupe aux Légumes de Maman (page 122)
Saumon à l'Unilatéral (page 99)
Mâche or endive salad
Grilled Pineapple with honey and goat cheese (page 117)
Glass of light red wine

GRANDMA LOUISE'S OATMEAL
WITH GRATED APPLE
Serves 2 to 4

When we visited my grandmother in snowy Alsace, she used to serve us this delicious and filling breakfast, rich in fiber and fruity nutrients. It is still one of my favorite winter breakfasts: true baby food for adults. My grandmother usually served her oatmeal variation with freshly baked brioche or kugelhopf (a wonderful cake with raisins and almonds that is one of the great specialties of Alsace). Today, I sometimes find it a filling meal unto itself, and I skip the bread. If I want a little more protein, I have a bite of cheese or some yogurt.

INGREDIENTS

1 cup old-fashioned oatmeal

2⅓ cups water

Pinch of salt

1 medium apple, coarsely grated

½ teaspoon lemon juice

⅓ cup milk

½ teaspoon butter

1. Combine the oatmeal, water, and salt in a medium saucepan. Bring to a boil.

2. Add the grated apple and lemon juice and cook for about 5 minutes, stirring occasionally.

3. Add the milk and butter. Stir well and cook for 1 minute. Serve immediately, perhaps with a sprinkle of brown sugar or a drizzle of maple syrup.

· ·

GRILLED PINEAPPLE

Serves 4

1. Make crisscross slashes with a knife on each slice of pineapple to get a nice presentation after grilling. Broil until the pineapple turns a nice caramel color, but be careful not to burn.

2. In a small saucepan, boil the lemon juice and honey for 2 to 3 minutes. Let cool, add pepper to taste, and drizzle over the pineapple slices. Serve immediately as is or with a scoop of verbena ice cream.

INGREDIENTS

4 1½-inch-thick slices of pineapple (fresh and ripe)

Juice of 2 lemons

2 teaspoons honey

Freshly ground pepper

N.B. IF YOU SERVE THIS DESSERT AT A WEEKEND LUNCH AFTER A BIG MIXED SALAD, YOU CAN REPLACE THE ICE CREAM WITH FRESH GOAT CHEESE OR RICOTTA. YOU WON'T HAVE THE SWEET-JUICY-PEPPERY COMBINATION, BUT THE PEPPERY ASPECT WILL BE MORE FORTHCOMING, AND THE CHEESE-PINEAPPLE PAIRING IS REFRESHINGLY DIFFERENT.

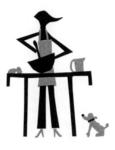

7

Seasonality (eating the best at its peak) and seasoning (the art of choosing and combining flavors to complement food) are vital for fighting off the food lover's worst enemy: not calories, but boredom. Eat the same thing in the same way time and again, and you'll need more just to achieve the same pleasure. (Think of it as "taste tolerance.") Have just one taste experience as your dinner (the big bowl of pasta, a big piece of meat), and you are bound to eat too much, as you seek satisfaction from volume instead of the interplay of flavor and texture that comes from a well-thought-out meal.

Playing with seasonality and seasoning is something most French women excel at. Many must also balance career and family. So it's not that they have so much more time than other women to dream up new creations every week; they just have a few more tricks up their sleeves. Just as French women have an uncanny knack for using the same scarf to create a different effect by draping it over the head, neck, shoulders, or waist, in the kitchen they master a few basic preparations and leave the rest to improvisation, the art of tweaking an old standby into seeming different. They do it by slightly altering the preparation or seasoning, by turning what is usually an entrée into an appetizer, or by transforming lunch leftovers into something rather different for several later meals. It's all about manipulating how the five senses are meeting what is put before them. And it can be as simple as choosing the more unusual yellow tomato over the standard red varieties. (Visual variety, color, and presentation are underestimated factors in food pleasure.) But you must think in terms of all the senses when planning meals. They are the reason why freshness, quality, and other sensations dictate how we feel about our food.

There are good and bad ways to "fool yourself" when it comes to eating. Many times our foods are not what they seem. Take sugar. It's not just in desserts anymore. It used to be a trick to add a little to tomato sauce, but nowadays most big assembly-line restaurants consider it mandatory. The same sweetening trend may be observed with balsamic vinegar. Ten years ago it was a rarity—as it should be, since true balsamic is scarce and expensive. But now that demand has soared, most restaurants freely use a cheap faux balsamic in which caramel and coloring conceal the absence of the flavors for which the real stuff is prized. Fat is another thing some restaurants lean on. If the ingredients aren't great, a bit more butter is a quick fix to make the dish taste better.

Despite its reputation as a butter-rich cuisine, authentic French cooking these days actually uses relatively little fat, preferring to create taste with other elements. And we are even stingier with sugar. But we get away with it only because we start with quality ingredients. Fresh, vine-ripened tomatoes naturally contain all the sweetness you should desire. But you can't fake a good tomato. Find what's good and in season where you are and work from there.

Now, how do we fool ourselves in a good way? We still want to *faire simple* (keep it simple). When I order in restaurants, I favor complicated, labor-intensive dishes. (I make a point, nevertheless, of asking the waiter how dishes are prepared. This simple form of interrogation requires no special expertise but can save hundreds of hidden calories per meal.) When I cook at home, however, as I do several times a week, I demand the most bang for the effort and the buck. Nothing delights me more than oohs and aahs over something literally thrown together with a few ingredients.

The following recipes are drawn mostly from my family experience. In each I aim to illustrate a way of eating simply but with satisfaction. I also indicate easy variations that can make the same dish seem very different or show how one dish can be used again as the basis for a subsequent meal. Cook once and eat for three days: it's a common principle.

How you serve a dish matters greatly. Some things offer enough sensory stimulation to stand virtually on their own, at least as the day's lighter meal; these need only some little accompaniments, a bit of bread, say. Others are interesting enough to be starters only, whetting the appetite rather than answering it decisively.

It matters whether or not you are serving the day's main meal. Again, in France, as in much of Europe, that's lunch. If you are having a full lunch with wine (which in France is sometimes employer subsidized via restaurant vouchers—*ah, la France!*), consider soups, our most versatile type of food. You might have a cup-size serving (nowadays more often served in a small well on a dinner plate) as the appetizer or between appetizer and entrée. (Remember, the French bourgeois meal as formalized in the eighteenth century was *potages,* hors d'oeuvres, *relevés de potage,* entrées, *rôti, entremets,* dessert, café, *pousse-café*! Few of us eat so many courses today.) If you're planning a big lunch, you might have a bowl of soup as the main part of dinner. This can be served with some bread and a bit of cheese. If dinner is the big meal, do soup or salad for lunch. Whether we eat the main meal of the day as lunch or dinner, the other meal is always a more modest affair.

SOUPS AND APPETIZERS

Each of these dishes can be used two ways. If it's the main event of the day's lighter meal, the portion can be increased somewhat. But if it's to be an appetizer for the day's main meal, always err on the side of too little. Many forget the literal meaning of "appetizer." Satisfaction is not a feeling you should be approaching after the first course of your day's main meal.

SOUPE AUX LÉGUMES DE MAMAN

Serves 8 to 12

In the summer we eat our soups chilled, in the winter piping hot. The theory goes that the French, who eat soup up to five times a week for dinner, eat better and less. We have a decent breakfast, a full lunch, and a less elaborate (but no less flavorful) dinner. The evening soup eater tends to consume less fat and less food overall, feeling satiated through the night, after which she needs "a real meal" on rising to get her through the morning.

We had a dozen variations on the vegetable soup theme, based on whatever was growing in the garden that season. My mother typically made vegetable soup on Thursdays for lunch, and as she had more time to cook that day, she would serve the soup with both potato pancakes (for the ladies in the family) and apple pancakes (which the men preferred). (Don't ask: My mother was always indulging the boys.) Her soup was judged "the best," according to my aunts and cousins, because of her final touches.

INGREDIENTS

2 potatoes
1 onion, peeled and quartered
2 garlic cloves, peeled
Salt and freshly ground pepper
4 leeks, white and tender green parts
1/2 small cabbage
3 celery ribs
2 turnips

1. Peel, wash, and roughly slice the potatoes. Place in a small pot and add water to cover. Add the quartered onion, garlic, salt, and pepper. Bring to a boil, reduce the heat, and simmer till tender (about 10 minutes). Drain and set aside.

2. Wash the remaining vegetables (except the tomatoes) and slice or dice them. Melt the 4 tablespoons of butter in a 15-quart stockpot and "sweat" the vegetables, stirring often (5 minutes). This procedure eliminates the more aggressive aromas of fresh vegetables.

3. Add the tomatoes, potatoes, onion, and garlic, and water to cover. Stir in the parsley, thyme, and bay leaves and continue to cook until all the vegetables are tender. Remove the bay leaves. Drain the vegetables, reserving the cooking liquid.

4. Purée the drained vegetables in a food mill, using the fine grating disk. Thin the soup with the reserved cooking liquid to the consistency you like (it shouldn't be too watery or too thick).

5. Correct the seasoning and add fresh herbs of your choice.

OPTIONAL FINISHING TRICKS:

Bring the soup to a boil. In a skillet, fry the thinly sliced onion in 1 tablespoon butter. Add to the soup. Add the crème fraîche, nutmeg, and salt to taste. Add pepper and serve immediately.

Alternatively, before putting the vegetables through the food mill, reserve 2 cups and add them to the soup just before serving. The "crunchy" vegetables will contrast with the velvety soup and will also force you to eat more slowly and thus satisfy you with less. This was the evening

4 carrots
4 tablespoons butter
2 cups canned (whole or chopped) tomatoes
2 sprigs of parsley
2 sprigs of fresh thyme
2 bay leaves

1 onion, peeled and thinly sliced
1 tablespoon butter
4 tablespoons crème fraîche
Pinch of freshly grated nutmeg
Salt and freshly ground pepper

version; the smooth lunch variant was accompanied with Mother's yummy pancakes.

You can also play a bit with different spices. Try ground cloves, cumin, or turmeric.

. . . .

Second service: Mother would save half of the soup before the finishing touch and serve it 2 days later, adding a sausage that she would sauté in a bit of oil and then stir into the soup. Voilà, another simple, filling, and nutritious evening meal made in a mere 15 minutes.

. . . .

COLD BEET
AND YOGURT SUMMER SOUP
Serves 4

This cold, thick soup was always a crowd-pleaser at my cousin's home in Provence. Easy to prepare, easy to serve, it's refreshing but also filling, with the yogurt furnishing protein and eliminating the need for a meat stock and even fish or meat later in the meal. Not only are the beets (with a season running from spring to fall) rich in fiber, but their brilliant color arrests the eyes. This recipe can be used as a summer dinner appetizer or as a main course at lunch.

INGREDIENTS

1. Mix the beets (they should be chunks that are a bit chewy and take a little more time to eat than if puréed) with the yogurt, shallots, cumin, salt, and pepper to taste. Refrigerate for 3 to 4 hours.

2. Serve the beets chilled in individual bowls and sprinkle with the dill. Served with a slice of bread and fruit (strawberries or melon) for dessert, this soup makes an excellent summer lunch.

4 medium beets, boiled till tender, then peeled and quartered

2 cups yogurt (page 151)

2 shallots, peeled and minced

Dash of cumin

Salt and freshly ground pepper

1 tablespoon minced fresh dill

CELERY ROOT RÉMOULADE

Serves 4

Celery root is used as the coleslaw of French cuisine, though it has a distinctive taste quite different from cabbage. Every French family and every decent bistro seems to have a different recipe. Often, celery root rémoulade is served along with a dish of grated carrots in a salad dressing. These raw veggies are a typical autumn or winter dish for an easy, delicious starter or colorful lunch en famille. Cooked celery root can also be used in soup, mixed with potatoes for a lovely, more refined "mash." Braised, the root (also known as celeriac) makes an excellent accompaniment for duck and game. Whenever we ate it raw, we always ate the carrots first and ended with the silky celery root.

INGREDIENTS

1 teaspoon mustard

1 tablespoon red wine vinegar

1 tablespoon lemon juice

1 tablespoon minced parsley

1 tablespoon minced cornichons

Salt and freshly ground pepper

½ cup mayonnaise

1 pound celery root, peeled, quartered, and shredded in a food processor; tossed with 1 teaspoon lemon juice to prevent discoloration

1. In a bowl, create the rémoulade (dressing) by mixing the mustard, vinegar, lemon juice, parsley, and cornichons. Season with salt and pepper to taste.

2. Mix in the mayonnaise and then the shredded celery root. Season to taste and refrigerate.

3. Take the celery root out of the refrigerator 20 minutes before serving and toss to fluff up. Serve with a slice of country bread.

N.B. YOU CAN SUBSTITUTE SOME MIXED HERBS OR FRESH CHERVIL AND TARRAGON FOR THE PARSLEY, BUT THEN IT WILL NO LONGER BE A CLASSIC VERSION.

· ·

LENTIL SOUP

Serves 4

For some reason, as kids we decided we didn't like lentils, but we loved leeks and sausages, so Tante Berthe *devised this trick to fool us.*

1. Pour the lentils in a stockpot and add 3 quarts water. Bring to a boil.

2. Add all the vegetables and seasonings. Cook for 1 hour.

3. At the end of the cooking time, slice the sausages into thick pieces and sauté in 1 tablespoon of the butter. Add to the lentils. Melt the remaining 1 tablespoon butter with the flour and add to the soup to thicken. Taste and correct the seasoning before serving.

INGREDIENTS

10 ounces lentils

4 ounces leeks, white part only, washed and minced

4 ounces celery, washed and minced

4 ounces carrots, washed and minced

1 onion studded with a clove

1 bay leaf

Salt and freshly ground pepper

4 Strasbourg sausages (high-quality hot dogs)

2 tablespoons butter

2 tablespoons flour

FINGERLINGS AND CAVIAR

Serves 4

Potatoes in France are serious business. There is a type for fries, another for mashing, one for roasting, and so on. It is nothing to see a dozen varieties for sale at a market. We would buy them in large bags and store them in the cellar. The only type we grew in the garden was the delicious charlotte, a small, succulent variety with a unique taste and firm flesh that Mother claimed suited caviar best. Caviar is pricey, but a little can really dress up some potatoes, especially for sudden guests. You can substitute salmon roe, domestic caviar, or simply minced chives.

INGREDIENTS

4 potatoes, fingerlings as an alternative to the French charlottes

6 ounces crème fraîche

Salt and freshly ground pepper

4 ounces caviar

1. Rinse the potatoes and cook in lightly salted water until cooked but not mushy. Drain and cut into 1-inch slices.

2. Season the crème fraîche to taste with the salt and pepper and dab on each potato slice. Garnish with the caviar. Serve immediately.

. . . .

RATATOUILLE
Serves 12

Another French classic as interpreted by my mother (based on a recipe from cousin Andrée in Aix-en-Provence) is something I still make today in the summer, when the variety of suitable vegetables is greatest. I can get three meals out of it. With almost no fat, the ratatouille seems rich, with the juice coming from the vegetables themselves. To get the most flavors, slow cooking is a must.

1. Use an equal amount of tomatoes, zucchini, and eggplant. Wash and cut into thick slices.

2. Using a large stockpot, make layers, starting with the eggplant, and then the tomatoes, and finally the zucchini. Repeat until the pot is filled almost to the brim. Add some garlic cloves and parsley sprigs between the layers. Season with salt and pepper.

3. Cover and cook over very low heat until the vegetables are tender, approximately 2 to 2½ hours.

4. Let cool, and serve 20 minutes later. Use soup bowls, since at this stage the ratatouille is more of a soup than a stew, with the liquid being mostly water from the veggies. Correct the seasoning and add a dash of extra-virgin olive oil and lots of freshly chopped parsley or basil or both.

INGREDIENTS

3 pounds tomatoes

3 pounds zucchini

3 pounds eggplant

12 garlic cloves

1 bunch of parsley (and/or basil)

Salt and freshly ground pepper

2 tablespoons extra-virgin olive oil

Freshly chopped parsley or basil, for garnish

The first version is served as a soup at room temperature.

The second version uses the leftovers as accompaniment to chicken or meat.

1. Warm up 2 tablespoons of olive oil and add the leftover ratatouille vegetables drained of their liquid (which can be reheated later and drunk lukewarm).

2. Cook over low to medium heat until the veggies have thickened.

3. Optional: Add ½ cup of grated cheese—Comté, Parmesan, or any variety you like.

The third version uses the leftover ratatouille from the second version as a pizza topping. It makes a good lunch or starter.

1. Buy or make pizza dough (with water, flour, yeast, and salt).

2. Beat 1 egg into the leftover ratatouille vegetables (a batch without the optional cheese) from the second version.

3. Spread the vegetable-egg mixture as a pizza topping on the pizza dough.

4. Add some freshly grated Parmesan and bake like a regular pizza.

. . . .

The name "main course" itself suggests one of the problems with the American notion of a meal. A "main" dish seems to be defined as the thing you have the most of. But eating a lot of any one element of a meal can be surprisingly less satisfying than eating equal portions of all things; as a result, the latter way is more "weight friendly." The key is to keep your eyes, your mouth, and your nose—your *mind*—entertained. A progression of "food-friendly" stimulation will reward you with contentment.

ZUCCHINI FLOWER OMELET

Serves 4

It never fails. During late spring–early summer, my shopping list for the open-air market in Manhattan's Union Square always includes zucchini flowers. I buy a few dozen, and invariably, a stranger in line asks what I do with them. It seems few people know, which perhaps explains why these vegetable flowers are so cheap. French and Italian women know lots of uses for them. I take them home for lunchtime omelets, a simple, balanced meal, yet impressive enough for entertaining.

INGREDIENTS

16 zucchini flowers

10 eggs

¼ cup water

Salt and freshly ground pepper

1 tablespoon butter

1 cup fresh goat cheese or fresh ricotta

Fresh herbs, for garnish

1. Wash the zucchini flowers and pat dry.

2. Beat together the eggs and water. Add the zucchini flowers to the egg mixture. Season with salt and pepper.

3. Melt the butter in a nonstick frying pan, and when piping hot add the zucchini-egg mixture. After a few minutes, when the eggs start setting, add the pieces of cheese all around. Continue to cook, but don't let the omelet get dry. Stop the cooking when it is still a bit runny. Garnish with fresh herbs and serve immediately.

· ·

ENDIVES WITH HAM
WITHOUT BÉCHAMEL SAUCE

Serves 4

This was another typical winter dish, whether for lunch on Saturday or dinner any night of the week, as Mother knew we would get our vegetables, protein, and fat all in one dish that was easy and not as costly to make as most other fish or meat dishes. And we all loved it. The sauce is something my mother called béchamel du sud *(compared with the classic béchamel sauce, this quick version made with tomato sauce is lighter and more digestible). A salad and piece of fruit complete the meal.*

1. Rinse the endives, cut bottoms, and cook in slightly salted water until tender. Drain.

2. Preheat the oven to 375 degrees. Wrap a slice of ham around each endive. Place in a baking dish. Pour the tomato sauce over the endives. Sprinkle the cheese on top and dot with the butter.

3. Put the gratin in the oven and bake for 20 minutes. Finish with 1 minute under the broiler to give it a nice brown top. Serve warm with country bread and a simple green salad.

INGREDIENTS

4 Belgian endives

Salt

4 slices of low-salt boiled ham

2 cups tomato sauce

2 ounces Swiss cheese, diced

2 ounces Parmesan cheese

1 tablespoon butter

. . . .

In springtime, you can prepare a similar dish using seasonal asparagus. You'll need about 5 asparagus stalks (enough to approximate the girth of the endive) per slice of ham.

. . . .

PORK CHOPS WITH APPLES

Serves 4

We had lots of apple trees of many varieties in our orchards, and the supply would last for the whole winter. Mostly I had them for a snack or in a dessert (as in Dr. Miracle's Apple Tart Without Dough), but here's one use in a main course that's a winner. It's incredibly easy yet nutritionally complete. I rather love mixing the sweet carb with the fat and protein in delicious defiance of current diet ideology.

INGREDIENTS

4 medium pork chops (you can substitute veal chops if you prefer)

4 whole cloves

½ cup dry white wine or vermouth

4 celery leaves

2 bay leaves

4 celery stalks, washed and finely diced

1 tablespoon butter

2 apples, cored and coarsely sliced

1 tablespoon brown sugar

4 ounces Swiss or Jarlsberg cheese, coarsely grated

1. Preheat the oven to 375 degrees. Butter a baking pan and place the pork chops in it.

2. Press a clove into each chop. Add the white wine, celery leaves, and bay leaves and put the pan in the preheated oven. Bake the chops for 30 minutes.

3. While the pork chops are baking, in a frying pan sauté the diced celery in the butter for 5 minutes, and then add the sliced apples and sprinkle with the brown sugar. Continue cooking over very low heat for 10 minutes, or until the apples are tender but not mushy.

4. Finish the pork chops by removing the bay and celery leaves and sprinkling the cheese over the top of each chop; baste and then broil for a few minutes to brown the top.

5. Serve the celery-apple mixture on the plate as an accompaniment to the pork chops. Use a few spoons of pan juices to further flavor the celery-apple mixture.

. . . .

To round out this meal, you can start with a consommé and end with a custard.

SNAPPER WITH ALMONDS

Serves 4

I didn't much care for fish when I was growing up, but I loved nuts. My mother knew both were essential for good nutrition, so she invented this way of slipping in the fish.

INGREDIENTS

½ cup toasted sliced almonds

2 tablespoons olive oil

2 tablespoons butter

4 snapper fillets (monkfish, halibut, or cod works, too), with skin, about 4 ounces each

Salt and freshly ground pepper

Juice of 1 lemon

½ cup chopped parsley

1. In a nonstick frying pan, toast the almonds over medium heat. Set aside.

2. Warm the olive oil and butter in the frying pan. Add the snapper skin-side up. Season with salt and pepper. Cook 4 minutes on each side. Transfer the fish to a warm serving plate and cover loosely with foil.

3. Add the lemon juice to the pan and whisk to blend with the pan juices. Pour over fillets, add the chopped parsley, and sprinkle with the toasted almonds. Serve immediately.

. . . .

We rarely ate only duck breasts at home because, like most people, we generally purchased an entire duck and prepared "our family version" of roast duck. But my oncle Charles came up with another recipe for his spa customers, using the relatively lean meat of the breasts only (the magret*), avoiding oil or butter in the preparation, and relying on the dry "marinade" for extra flavor. Calling it Gasconne was a subtle way of fooling his guests. Most were wealthy Parisians who had never set foot in Gascony, a region in the southwest of France known for its ducks and geese and,* naturellement, *great duck dishes. So before tasting even a morsel of this relatively light preparation, they were psychologically primed for the heights of Gasconne delicacy.*

1. In a large baking pan, mix the salt, bay leaves, thyme, parsley, garlic, shallot, and peppercorns. Roll the *magrets* in the mixture and spread them out in the pan skin-side up.

2. Cover with plastic wrap and refrigerate the breasts for 24 hours, turning them once.

3. Remove the *magrets* from the marinade. Wipe or rinse the *magrets* to remove excess seasoning; pat them dry with paper towels. (Discard the marinade.) Arrange the breasts skin-side down on a broiler rack and place under the broiler 4 inches away from the heat. Broil 2 minutes; turn them

INGREDIENTS

Pinch of coarse salt

Pinch of crumbled dried bay leaves

Pinch of crumbled dried thyme leaves

1 teaspoon chopped parsley

2 garlic cloves, peeled and sliced

½ teaspoon finely diced shallot

8 black peppercorns, coarsely crushed

4 duck *magrets* (breasts)

over and broil 3 to 4 minutes. Depending on the size and thickness of the *magrets*, the broiling time may need to be increased. The *magrets* should be medium-rare.

4. Transfer the *magrets* to a carving board and let rest 2 to 3 minutes. Thinly slice the breast meat crosswise on the bias and serve.

. . . .

SALAD OF DUCK À L'ORANGE

Serves 4

Use leftovers from the Duck à la Gasconne recipe that have been refrigerated.

1. Peel the oranges. Cut off the skin and white pith. Slice off and remove the membrane that separates the wedges.

2. Make the dressing by mixing the Dijon mustard with the red wine vinegar and the olive oil.

3. Toss the salad greens, shallots, green beans, and orange slices with the dressing. Spoon onto individual plates.

4. Cut the duck breasts on the bias into ½-inch strips and arrange on the salad greens. Drizzle some olive oil on the duck breasts. Serve with a slice of olive bread.

INGREDIENTS

2 seedless oranges

1 teaspoon Dijon mustard

3 tablespoons red wine vinegar

6 tablespoons olive oil plus additional for drizzling

½ pound salad greens (mesclun mixed with arugula or red oak lettuce with frisée)

2 teaspoons minced shallots

½ pound green beans, trimmed and blanched

2 cooked *magrets* (breasts) (bring to room temperature while you prepare the salad)

TAGLIATELLE WITH LEMON

Serves 4

Life without pasta? Perish the thought. It's not a French thing per se, pota-toes being the more ubiquitous starch of choice. But in Alsace, noodles are served with lots of dishes, from fish to game, mostly with heavy sauces somewhat like those from the Piedmont region of Italy. We had pasta a few times a month when I was a kid, but we tended to favor the lighter, more intensely flavored preparations, like this cream-and-lemon combination Tante Caroline developed. She considered it a perfect lunch staple accom-panied by a salad and piece of fruit. Her daughter, Louise, tells me it's still very popular with all the kids. Pay attention to the portions!

INGREDIENTS

12 ounces tagliatelle
4 lemons
1 tablespoon olive oil
6 ounces crème fraîche
4 ounces Parmesan cheese
Salt and freshly ground pepper

1. Cook the tagliatelle in boiling salted water until al dente. Drain.

2. While the pasta is cooking, grate the zest of lemons and squeeze and reserve the juice of 1 lemon.

3. In a saucepan, warm up the olive oil, add the zest, and cook over low flame for 2 minutes. Add the crème fraîche and bring to a boil; pour in the reserved lemon juice and bring to a boil again.

4. When the cream starts to thicken, add the Parmesan, season to taste, mix well, and cook for another minute. Add the drained pasta and toss to mix. Serve immediately.

Pasta is good for you, but not eaten (as in America) as a main dish, in huge portions. Italians have it as a first or second course before the main course. Don't imagine you'll lose weight eating a big bowl with a dull tomato sauce—you'll never reach contentment. Add some fresh ricotta, a few pieces of tuna or veal or any meat, and less will seem like more. The French love pasta, but they love it with less fat. Among the standard preparations are a tomato coulis with onion and thyme or a basil sauce with garlic and a few pine nuts. Each includes 1 tablespoon of olive oil per person, and the dish is further "moistened" with 2 to 3 tablespoons of the pasta water. Then a dusting of Parmesan, sparingly, as in Italy. Net intake is about 3 ounces per person, but followed by fish or meat.

The French seem to have a broader notion of dessert than Americans do. American desserts tend to be rich and heavy, frequently defeating the goals of balance and eating in moderation. They are also much sweeter on average, which is very much a matter of conditioned expectation. In France, we would not have such a dessert following other rich courses. It's more appropriate when the preceding fare is lighter. By the same token, not having room for dessert would suggest that the preceding parts of the meal have been too large or too rich. In any case, forcing dessert on a full stomach is never a good idea. Balance your dessert with what comes before. And develop a taste for things that aren't supersweet, like cheese and fruit. The elaborate pastries—including my beloved *mille-feuille*—are eaten more as occasional tea cakes than at the end of a meal.

When it comes to dessert, permit me to offer two restaurant tactics. The first you probably know: sharing, especially ordering one for two. But if everyone's ordering her own and you don't want to be a drag, try this: Take a few bites very slowly, until others are almost done. Then tell a story or talk to your neighbor. While you're talking, others keep eating; meanwhile, discreetly put your utensils in the five o'clock "done" position; when the server comes to collect your plate, everyone will still be listening to your story and won't notice your subtle moderation. I have done this so many times, and it always works.

POACHED PEARS

Serves 4

1. In a heavy saucepan, bring the wine and sugar to a boil. Lower the heat and simmer for 5 more minutes.

2. Add the lemon juice and pears. Cook for 10 minutes over medium to low flame. Cool and refrigerate.

3. Bring the pears to room temperature before serving. Add 1 scoop of vanilla ice cream to each serving.

INGREDIENTS

2 cups Muscat Beaumes de Venise

½ cup sugar

2 tablespoons lemon juice

4 Bosc pears, peeled, cored, and halved

4 scoops of vanilla ice cream

. . . .

For extra luxury, serve each pear in a little pool of melted dark chocolate.

. . . .

BAKED APPLES

Serves 4

In the good old days, autumn meant apples and nuts piling up from our orchard. Luckily, my mother knew countless ways of using them. It's one of the true pleasures of the season, biting into a fresh apple before it's had a chance to dehydrate or grow mealy. Fortunately, distribution of apples in season has greatly improved in the United States, and good apples move fast enough that even a better supermarket may prove a good source. The crunch of a good apple following a meal may furnish just the right counterpoint to the preceding textures. (Remember, it's not just our stomach, but our mouth too that we need to satisfy. Sometimes compulsive eating is more a nervous urge simply to ingest and to chew than actual hunger.) And they are easy on the calorie count. As kids, we always preferred cooked apples to raw, so especially on those days when she was serving a soup or entrée less popular with the kids, my mother made sure to motivate us with this dessert, which seemed much more luxurious than it was. She'd also make delicious applesauce that was served as a little snack when we came back from school.

INGREDIENTS

⅓ cup chopped walnuts

4 apples (Cortland, Golden Delicious, or Rome Beauty)

4 teaspoons butter

4 teaspoons sugar mixed with ½ teaspoon cinnamon

2 tablespoons water

1. Place the walnuts on a baking sheet and toast them in a 250-degree oven for about 5 minutes, until they are fragrant. Set aside.

2. Wash and core the apples. Place them in a baking dish. Combine the butter, sugar-cinnamon mixture, and toasted walnuts.

3. Fill the cavity of each apple with the mixture, dividing it evenly among the 4 apples. Pour the water into the bottom of the baking dish.

4. Bake the apples at 375 degrees for 30 minutes. Serve warm. You can make the dessert more festive by pouring 1 teaspoon of heavy cream over each apple just before serving, garnishing with a sprig of mint for color, or placing an edible flower on the side.

. . . .

FLOATING ISLAND
WITH A DOSE OF COCOA POWDER
Serves 4 to 6

The French rarely eat eggs for breakfast and don't drink milk by itself, but we consume plenty of both, mostly in sauces and desserts. (Of course, we eat eggs in omelets, but these are served for lunch or dinner.) In one classic dessert, les oeufs à la neige *(eggs with snow), known in restaurants by the fancier name* île flottante *(floating island), we get plenty of eggs, milk, protein, and fat with limited carbohydrates. And as rich desserts go, this one isn't so fattening because much of the egg component is egg white. You'll find it attractive, delectable, and easy. My mother would often make it in the evening and serve it the next day at lunch. Since it was among my favorite desserts, when I'd see her prepare it, I knew that the next day's menu would include something good for me that I did not like. "Eat it all and you can have dessert," she'd say. Several times a month, I was shamelessly bought with a floating island.*

INGREDIENTS

2½ cups whole milk

⅔ cup plus 1 tablespoon sugar

1 teaspoon pure vanilla extract

4 eggs

¼ teaspoon salt

Cocoa powder for sprinkling

1. Scald the milk in a large, heavy-bottomed saucepan. Add ⅓ cup of the sugar and the vanilla. Cover and remove from heat.

2. Separate the eggs and reserve the egg yolks in a mixing bowl.

3. In another bowl, beat the whites with the salt until foamy and then gradually beat in the 1 tablespoon of sugar. Beat the egg whites to stiff peaks. (An electric mixer is handy here.)

4. Return the saucepan with milk to the heat and bring to a boil. Reduce the heat to low.

5. With a soup spoon, scoop out a mound of the egg whites and drop into the milk. Cook gently for 2 minutes and turn gently to cook the other side for 2 minutes. Remove and drain on a dry towel. Let cool, then cover and refrigerate on a plate until ready to serve.

6. In the bowl containing the egg yolks, gradually beat in the remaining 1/3 cup of sugar and continue beating for 2 to 3 minutes until the mixture is pale yellow and forms a ribbon. Gradually add the hot milk in a thin stream to slowly warm up the yolks and avoid scrambling them. Chill the custard in a serving bowl.

7. When ready to serve, place the poached egg whites on top of the custard. Provide a bowl of cocoa powder for each guest to sprinkle over the whites (we kids were allowed the dose of our dreams!).

. . . .

When this dessert was served at our formal Sunday lunches to guests, my mother would add 1 tablespoon of rum to the custard and either drizzle caramel on the whites or grate over some dark chocolate. (I preferred the latter, finding the caramel too sweet, as I still do.)

. . . .

Yogurt remains my secret weapon. Ever since Dr. Miracle first prescribed two servings a day, it's been a no-brainer snack and dessert. But full adoration did not bloom until I visited Crete.

We did not eat much yogurt at home when I was growing up. We preferred *petits suisses,* a soft white cheese that we would sprinkle with cocoa powder. We did not drink raw milk, either, except during the summers in the country at my grandmother's house. She kept cows, and every evening before going to bed, we had to drink *un bol* (the breakfast big bowl) of fresh milk, still warm from the source. At home, we also had our "dairy" requirement via custard, flan, crème anglaise, pudding, and all the warm savory dishes, mostly served in winter, using milk as a cooked ingredient.

Yogurt is actually better for you than any of these dairy products. Doctors typically recommend that patients on antibiotics—destroyers of intestinal flora—eat one serving with each meal. One gram of basic yogurt has something like ten million live bacteria *Lactobacillus bulgaricus* and *Streptococcus thermophilus,* vital to your digestive well-being.

For me yogurt took a little getting used to. The fruit and fillings didn't exist in those days. Given my diagnosed sweet tooth, the classic *yaourt nature* was not immediately a palatable substitute for dessert. So Dr. Miracle said I could add ½ teaspoon of honey or a sprinkle of wheat germ. In the spring, a moderately sweetened rhubarb compote spiked with cinnamon worked well, as did a mix of succulent strawberries or raspberries. There were days when I had nothing in my pantry to add (following his tip not to stock offenders), and that's when I started surrendering to the pleasures of plain yogurt. Nothing tastes quite like it, that combination of tartness and creaminess.

While still a student, I would travel in Greece on five dollars a day during the summer. I had studied modern Greek, so I liked to stay at homes and practice speaking with natives. The furnishings were spartan, rarely more than a shower and a bed (and more often a mattress laid on the terrace roof, as this was the high season and many families would take in several foreign students). Since I spoke the language, however, the astonished family often spoiled me with a bed. Sometimes they wouldn't even charge me, but always they would invite me into their kitchen in the morning for a glass of water, a demitasse of that very strong "Greek coffee" (called Turkish in most other places) . . . and a yogurt.

One summer in Crete, I stayed with the kindly and petite wife of a sea captain; she told me that when he was away, she practically lived on yogurt and fruit except for a small piece of fish and some greens at dinner. Skipping the cheap, greasy tavernas, I started going to the tiny grocery stores near the beach and would buy my lunch—yogurt and a peach. The peaches were perfectly in season: luscious and with an almost liquory juiciness. After ten days following her program—walking and swimming each day—I left Crete floating in my clothes (I later discovered I had lost three pounds yet have rarely felt so pampered since).

Of course, nothing equals a yogurt from Crete, made with goats' milk. I've learned that the island's entire food chain is rich in alpha-linolenic acid, present in all the edible wild plants. Cretan women still pick various herbs and plants, and since the livestock feed themselves, poultry, eggs, and milk contain two or three times more of that beneficial nutrient.

Even some French store-bought yogurt contains the host of undesirable ingredients you find in the American versions—artificial preservatives, colors, flavorings, sugar, and other sweeteners. So in Crete I made sure to learn from the captain's wife how to make my own.

It requires some starter—either a commercially available combination of live bacteria cultures or simply a spoonful of good store-bought yogurt, provided it contains active cultures—and a yogurt machine, one of the best minor investments I've ever made.

Here is the recipe: quick and easy . . . the machine does the work.

HOMEMADE YOGURT
WITH A YOGURT MAKER

1. Warm up the milk in a saucepan over medium-low heat until bubbles appear around the edge and steam rises from the surface. Remove the saucepan from heat and insert a thermometer stirrer. When the temperature reaches 110 to 115 degrees, add the starter to one of the jars. Add some of the heated milk and stir until well blended. Pour the mixture back into the saucepan, a little at a time, stirring well.

2. Fill all 8 jars, cover securely with lids, and place the jars into the "machine" (which is really a temperature-controlled warmer) and follow the cooking instructions. It will take 6 to 10 hours (easy to do overnight), depending on the tartness and firmness desired.

3. When done, chill the jars in the refrigerator for a few hours before serving. You can keep the yogurt for up to 2 weeks in the fridge.

INGREDIENTS

1 quart whole or 2 percent milk

1 tablespoon plain yogurt as a starter or 1 tablespoon of a commercial starter culture (available at natural food stores)

Yogurt maker with cooking thermometer (I use the Donvier brand with eight jars)

If you don't want to invest in a yogurt maker, here's a foolproof, centuries-old recipe of which I was recently reminded by a taxi driver on the Greek island of Mykonos. Greek taxi drivers are something else: extroverted, educated, multilingual, knowledgeable, memorable, and opinionated. I forget what question we had asked him, but it launched him on a discourse about life, gardening, importing ladybugs from Holland, family, hotels, the comparative merits of restaurants on the island, and eventually yogurt.

HOMEMADE YOGURT
WITHOUT A YOGURT MAKER

1. Warm up the milk in a saucepan over medium-low heat until bubbles appear around the edge and steam rises from the surface.

2. Pour the warm milk into a large bowl to cool until the temperature reaches 110 to 115 degrees on a cooking thermometer. If you don't have a thermometer, do what the locals do: the temperature is correct when you can keep your index finger in the warm milk for 20 seconds.

3. Put the starter in a small bowl, add some of the heated milk, and stir until well blended. Return the mixture to the large bowl, a third at a time, making sure to stir and blend well after each addition. End with a final stir, making sure all is well blended. Cover with a heavy towel and keep in a warm place 6 to 8 hours or overnight (a gas oven with a pilot light is fine, or placing a saucepan of hot water in the oven to raise the temperature will help if your home is not warm enough).

4. When set, cover the bowl with plastic wrap and refrigerate for 8 hours before serving. If thicker yogurt is desired, empty chilled yogurt in a muslin bag or cheesecloth, suspend over a bowl, and drain.

INGREDIENTS

1 quart whole or 2 percent milk

1–2 tablespoons plain yogurt as a starter or 1–2 tablespoons of a commercial starter culture (available at natural food stores)

8

LIQUID ASSETS

EAU DE VIE

Scarcely anyone who has gone to American schools hasn't learned that water is the essence of life. Recently we spent close to $1 billion to discover whether or not there was ever water on Mars. Why? Because without water, life as we know it could never have existed there. And we wouldn't long exist here on Earth if we quit drinking. Water makes up 70 percent of our body weight, 80 percent of our blood, 70 percent of our lean muscle, and a whopping 85 percent of our gray matter, which perhaps suggests why dehydrated people become delirious long before their other bodily functions give out. Given these facts, which are far more certain than most "scientific" claims made in diet books, it's something of a mystery why

Americans don't drink more water, particularly since, as any French woman knows, it's a powerful way of controlling one's weight, virtually without sacrifice. In fact, if you simply drank four or five more glasses per day, it would be extremely difficult not to lose some weight over time.

As in all matters, pleasure is a key to understanding the Franco-American divide. Most American women quench their thirst with soft drinks, coffee, juices, and perhaps some tea. These are all mostly water, true, but some, especially the ones containing caffeine, are also diuretic, promoting a bit of water to be lost even as you consume some. There is simply no way of getting enough water unless you drink it straight, but it would seem that most Americans take no pleasure in pure water. They prefer something with some added taste—even if it's the taste of coffee left sitting all day on the burner or the aftertaste of diet sodas. Still, most women know they should drink more water, so they typically compromise by having a couple of glasses a day in addition to their other soft beverages. But they are only fooling themselves, and not in the good way. So, too, are those who tote around their bottle of Evian but really take just a few sips; they're not getting even close to what their bodies need to stay hydrated and to flush out toxins and the wastes of metabolism. If you want to see what water means to your skin, try adding a little to a shrunken dry sponge.

Most people don't take into account how much water we lose passively, especially in very hot or cold weather. Perspiration is an obvious debit, but in frigid dry air, we are losing a great deal through our skin and breath. The body is not a watertight sac; the skin absorbs, but mostly surrenders, water. All told, we lose about ten to twelve cups of water a day (even when we sleep) through breathing, perspiration, and body wastes. As you can see, even the widely recommended eight glasses a day may result in a deficit, depending on the size of your glass. The key to health and to harnessing the weight-loss power of water is not radical: just consume a bit more than you lose.

In my New York office, we have a cooler with a big inverted jug, which our maintenance man keeps supplied. He once confessed to me that his life is easier when I am not around. Since I hardly give him any work, I was puzzled. He explained with a mischievous grin, "It's the water bottles, ma'am. When you travel it lasts a week, but when you're here I have to change it every other day." That made it clear to me that our staff were parched by their own hands. All day long, our able-bodied crew (mostly women, but we apparently have some male camels, too) have no trouble running down to the deli to buy coffee or soft drinks. But rarely do I see any of them at the water cooler, the proverbial American gathering point for goofing off.

The contrast with our Paris headquarters couldn't be more stark. Each day a one-liter bottle of water is distributed to each office and cubicle, and if that's not enough (and it isn't!), there's a room always filled with them, where anyone can go to get more. When we have meetings, bottles are set up all over the conference room. Not in America. Even the small bottles on the conference table remain mostly untouched after a few hours, though the coffee urn is emptied and the cans of Diet Coke vanish.

And it isn't just an office affair. I've stayed at lots of homes all across the United States and noticed that a single water bottle in the fridge can easily remain at the same level for days, while sodas, beer, and all kinds of sugary drinks get consumed by the economy size. Needless to say, children who don't see their parents drink water are not likely to develop the habit on their own.

When I am in France and visit young relatives, I still see what I recognize from my own childhood. Everyone starts the day with a glass of water. At every meal, there is always a big bottle of mineral water on the table. People help themselves throughout the day—and it isn't kept in the fridge. (Sometimes water aversion is actually an understandable distaste for suffering the shock of something cold. You might find water at room temperature much easier on your throat and teeth, not to mention your stomach.)

French people don't drink tap water; ours usually doesn't taste good enough to drink. Some American water aversion is rooted in a commonsense reluctance to buy what one imagines should flow free. The great variety of bottled water may seem effete to some. Even in American cities, there are dozens of brands on the shelf. It may seem just one more thing to lug and obviously more expensive than what flows from the tap. In fact, you may be perfectly fine drinking what comes out of your faucet, but if you're not having your share, you need to ask why.

In our house, the still waters (*eaux plates*) of choice were Vittel and Volvic, and the only sparkling (*gazeuse*) brand for us was and remains Badoit. We were hooked ages ago by an alliterative old jingle that ran *"Et badadit et badadoit, la meilleure eau c'est la Badoit."* We've tried others, but the acquired taste wins out every time.

The French are the world's number two sparkling water drinkers (after the Italians). We prefer *l'eau plate,* but even without fizz the choices are vast. At Colette, a restaurant in Paris (actually a store with an underground restaurant and bar), you can taste between eighty and one hundred types of water from all over the world. Water drinking has become so fancy that there is now a word for the related connoisseurship— aquanomy—and water has its *crus,* tastes, and vocabulary; one variety is distinguished from another according to the levels of calcium and magnesium and other mineral characteristics.

In case you were wondering, American mineral waters are considered bland. Could this hint at why almost two-thirds of the population is chronically dehydrated? Perhaps, but it surely must explain in part why we import so much water not only from France and Italy, but from dozens of other countries. It amuses me in American restaurants to be routinely offered water from Fiji—an "artesian" variety.

It could be that such delicacy about water simply goes against the American grain. Nevertheless, it's time we face up to the most widespread deficiency in consumption habits. And weight control is a good motivation, if not the most urgent.

For one thing, we have to understand that the thirst sensation can often be mistaken for hunger: very often when we have *un petit creux* or *une petite faim,* we have in fact *une petite soif.* So we confuse a little thirst for a little hunger, not surprising if we're drinking too little and are overdependent on the water content of our food. For the same reason, water is a potent *coupe faim*—hunger buster. Regularly filling your stomach with it promotes feelings of contentment and also eases butterflies.

I have my own theories about getting enough. I do carry a bottle in my bag, but it's more of an *en-cas,* not my daily supply. To get the maximum benefit, you need to drink water all day long. I have a glass when I get up, one before bed, and lots in between. I always have one thirty minutes or so before each meal (I don't need to remind myself anymore; it becomes automatic very quickly), and I avoid drinking water with my meals, as it slows down digestion. (I do, however, recommend water with meals during your recasting and stabilization phases: what's lost in digestive speed is well compensated for in calorie-free volume.) Sparkling water, on the other hand, is a matter of personal preference, of course, depending on the state of your digestive tract, which is not always in the mood for additional gas. Personally, I have it only occasionally, getting my share of bubbles from Champagne, which has its own rewards. But in summer, I do find a glass of sparkling water with a dash of fresh lemon juice to be wonderfully refreshing. And, of course, I love a *citron pressé* at my favorite café on the boulevard St. Germain.

The wonderful thing about water, apart from its total lack of calories, is that for all practical purposes you can't have too much. It's essential to all body functions, and even the business of getting rid of it is good for you, flushing out contaminants and preventing mineral deposits. (If you've ever had a kidney stone, I am told, you'll never skimp on water again.) Water also helps maintain the electrolyte balance in our bodies and can ease everything from muscle cramps (ever heard of those?) to headaches, weakness, and fatigue. And let's not forget *les coups de vieux.* Water is my lubricant par excellence, restoring my body and soul. Adding water will do more for your complexion than all the high-tech rejuvenating molecules you can pack into a jar. If there is a fountain of youth, it's flowing with pure H_2O. So make friends with water.

Through healthy eating, you can get about 40 percent of the water you need from food, but only by eating a good variety of fruits and vegetables. (Not much water in that rib-eye steak.) The rest is up to you, so bottoms up. Sample various mineral waters to see if one is especially to your taste. (Remember Tim Robbins in *The Player,* ordering a different brand in every scene!) If tap is your preference, invest in a purifier or filter. (Remember, the French consider their tap water nonpotable, and even the finest municipal reservoir could use some help in the taste department.) Finally, wherever you can, increase liquids that do not deplete body water. I prefer soups, herbal teas (don't personally care for the green variety despite its miraculous properties), even milk and diluted fresh fruit juices in moderation.

In France, coffee is usually reserved for breakfast and the end of a meal. We don't drink it all day long as some Americans do; that's an awful habit. If you're not having water before your first cup, you'll start the day in the red, as the caffeine drains your water reserves (which have already been depleted during sleep). Tea drinking is still not a big thing for the French (perhaps that has something to do with British relations over the centuries). While I do notice more tea salons (black tea), I fear their job is mainly to lure tourists looking for another place to eat pastry! Tisanes (herbal teas brewed from a vast variety of plants—anything except the tea leaf) are what we enjoy both at home and in restaurants. With little or no caffeine, they are almost as good as pure water, and they have been part of our gastronomic repertoire for ages, drunk mostly after dinner or before bedtime.

In my home, we were all addicted to herbal teas. Maybe it was my mother's trick to make sure we'd all drink water before bedtime, but I also remember it as a sensory pleasure. Just after dinner during the week and later on weekends, brewing and sharing a fragrant pot was a family ritual, the day's final excuse to draw together. I loved to pick the tisane. There were always six to ten glass jars filled with the dried herbs we had either picked in the forest behind my grandmother's house in Alsace or else brought back from summer holidays in Provence. From my grandmothers and aunts I learned a wealth of home remedies: *verveine* (verbena, with its lemon-citrus flavor) and *tilleul* (from the linden tree and noted for its hint of woodiness) for any time, but particularly after a meal; *camomille* (a floral aroma with an applelike taste) was for sleep; *menthe* (mint), which is served all the time in Morocco (probably brought back as a colonial custom), would help digestion; and so on. Sometimes we'd concoct our own aromatic blends and bundle them into sachets, alongside which the bleached supermarket teabags of today seem pathetically sterile and inert.

As we sipped the last beverage of the night, we'd usually talk about our plans for the next day or something interesting someone had read or heard; it was a fifteen-minute social ritual during the week, but on weekends and invariably when we had guests, it could last a couple of hours. No munching, just sipping. I particularly remember when I was a student in Paris coming home once a month; my mother and I would be the last ones up, talking till two or three in the morning over a few cups of tisanes . . . and then sleeping like angels.

Vivre de pain, d'amour, et d'eau fraîche, goes the French saying: Live on bread, love, and fresh water. It doesn't get more basic than that.

Water, as I say, must be taken in slowly throughout the day. Soups are a great way to get it into our bodies and terrifically satisfying in relation to their calories. We French are probably the biggest soup eaters in the world. When I was growing up, it was often the evening staple. Since we'd have the day's main meal at lunch, dinner was limited to *une assiette de soupe* and a piece of cheese or a soft-boiled egg or a small green salad and then a fruit. Soups were a serious matter. They were all homemade in *le plus grand pot,* which could be good news or bad, depending on which soup it was, since the "aromas" would fill the house all day.

One of my favorites was chicken, to which we would add alphabet pastina. Yvette, our *nounou,* dreaded the endless dinners when we lingered, making words in the soup dish. She'd try to move us along: *"Mange ta soupe."* Good advice, actually. *Vermicelle* was another favorite, and so was the vegetable soup, which of course varied with the season. Soup was a wonderful staple, particularly in winter, when it warmed us up. There were others, too, the ones children don't usually like; and Yvette had to find tricks to make us enjoy them. Carrot soup wasn't bad, but soups of lentils, spinach, leeks, or cabbage— their funny smells infusing the kitchen (where we had all our meals except Sunday lunch)—turned us off. Eating the soup after smelling it all day was a trial for us kids, though not the adults. Yvette would make up elaborate stories to distract us, and just as she was getting to the good part, she'd say, *"Mange la soupe,"* compelling a few more spoonfuls before she would continue. In the worst-case scenario—definitely the cabbage soup, which we called *la soupe des paysans* (peasant soup)—the promise of a treat afterward was the only effective way to get us to empty our dishes. It was tough training us (poor Yvette: her boyfriend was waiting for her, but she never knew when she'd leave the house). By the time we were teenagers, however, we'd become proper French citizens, eating all these soups, even the smelly ones, with pleasure. Making a regular place for soup in your diet is better learned as a child, but if you can do it now, you'll benefit from one basic secret of French women. If I had to pick one soup from childhood that I loved, it would be the *soupe aux légumes* (vegetable soup) that my mother would make for lunch in the winter maybe twice a month. It was paired with potato or apple pancakes.

BASIC VEGETABLE SOUP

Serves 8

My mother cooked all the vegetables in water. Although potatoes were always included, the choice of other vegetables was often a matter of availability.

INGREDIENTS

2 potatoes (about 4 ounces each)

1 small cabbage

2 leeks

2 carrots

2 celery ribs with their leaves

2 medium-size yellow onions

Freshly ground pepper

2 teaspoons salt

½ teaspoon dried thyme

2 bay leaves

Small bunch of fresh parsley

10 cups of water

1. Peel the vegetables. Cut the potatoes and cabbage into small cubes; wash the leeks carefully and slice them crosswise. Slice the carrots and celery as well, and quarter the onions. You should have about 10 cups of prepared vegetables. Use the same amount of water.

2. Place all the vegetables in a stockpot. Season with a grind of fresh pepper, add the salt, thyme, bay leaves, and parsley, and toss with the vegetables. Add the water. Cover and bring to boil slowly. Reduce the heat and simmer for 1½ hours.

3. Remove and discard the bay leaves. Drain the vegetables, reserving the cooking liquid. Purée the vegetables in a food mill, using the cooking liquid to thin them out, if necessary. Reheat the soup to the boil. Taste and correct the seasonings and serve.

. . . .

At the end of the fall, Mother would add the last tomatoes of the garden and in the dead of winter half of a celery root, but you can add whatever you like. Same for herbs—suit your fancy.

. . . .

QUICK AND EASY CARROT SOUP

Serves 4

1. Place the carrots in a pot with an equal amount of boiling water. Cook until al dente, about 15 minutes.

2. Purée the soup in a food mill. Season to taste with a pinch of sugar, salt, and pepper. Just before serving, add a dollop of butter and some fresh dill or coriander.

INGREDIENTS

5 cups peeled and sliced carrots

Pinch sugar

Salt

Freshly ground pepper

1 dollop butter

Fresh dill or coriander, to garnish

FANCY CREAM OF CARROT SOUP

Serves 8

INGREDIENTS

2 bay leaves

5 cups peeled and
sliced carrots

4 medium-size onions,
peeled and sliced

2 potatoes, peeled
and sliced

1 tablespoon sugar

2 tablespoons heavy cream

Salt and freshly ground
pepper

Whole nutmeg

1. Bring 10 cups of water to a boil. Add the bay leaves and all the vegetables. Simmer for 45 minutes.

2. Remove the bay leaves, and then purée the carrots in a food mill. Add the sugar and heavy cream and heat over low flame until piping hot. Season to taste with salt and pepper. Grate a pinch of nutmeg as garnish.

SOUPE EXOTIQUE

Serves 4

1. Combine 1½ cups of the milk with the ground almonds and set aside to infuse for 30 minutes. Mix, put through a sieve, and add the almond extract.

2. Clean the haricots verts and add to a pot of lightly salted boiling water. Cook for 8 minutes. Drain. Rinse under cold water and purée in a food processor with the remaining cup of milk. Add the vinegar and correct the seasoning. Set aside.

3. Peel and cut the mango and purée in a food processor with the lime juice and a pinch of freshly grated nutmeg. Set aside.

4. Combine the almond-milk mixture with the puréed haricots verts and serve it at room temperature in a soup dish. Drizzle the mango mixture over the top and add salt and pepper to taste.

INGREDIENTS

2½ cups 2 percent milk

1 cup finely ground almonds

¼ teaspoon bitter almond extract

1 pound haricots verts (thin string beans)

1 tablespoon red wine vinegar

Half of a very ripe mango

1½ tablespoons fresh lime juice

Freshly grated nutmeg

Salt and freshly ground pepper

N.B. STEPS 1 TO 3 CAN BE PREPARED IN ADVANCE. FOR A THINNER CONSISTENCY, USE FEWER ALMONDS AND MORE MILK, OR USE HALF MILK, HALF WATER.

Faites simple (Keep it simple), advised Escoffier, and every great cook learns to do just that. The master was most likely referring to solid food, but by my lights, the rule should also cover liquid food, which is how the French regard wine. It has calories; it has nutrients; it has flavors. Its potential as an intoxicant doesn't loom large in our thinking (or drinking), as most French consider wine a sacred gift, to be enjoyed but not abused. The French poet Baudelaire said that if wine were to disappear from human production, there would be a void in human health and intelligence, and that void would be worse than all the excesses it's guilty of. We drink wine not to dull our senses, but to awaken them. And it is vitally important to our enjoyment of food.

My mother, who taught me from an early age to value simplicity in all things, never served any aperitif but Champagne. Her reasoning was simple. Hard liquor requires a bar, special paraphernalia, and a variety of glasses, as well as messy shaking or stirring. More important, it numbs more than it tickles the taste buds. When you've spent time and money preparing delicious food for your guests, the last thing you want is to render them unable to taste it. That will eliminate one of the most important topics of conversation!

These days, after years of steady growth in wine appreciation, I notice a competing trend among Americans: a renaissance of hard liquor drinking. At restaurants it's common, especially among the young, to order something hard while waiting at the bar and then continue with the same drink over dinner. The alcohol content of such beverages can be three to four times greater than that of the same amount of wine, so you are getting vastly more calories together with a duller sense of taste. Also dulled is your natural sense of contentment, and you invariably eat more. Maybe it's the key to how some restaurants survive serving mediocre food. (It's certainly true that profit margins on booze are much higher than those on food.)

If you haven't already been converted to the pleasures of wine, you have deprived your taste buds of a world of flavors and perhaps left yourself vulnerable to seeking compensation with too much food. Wine is not only the perfect accompaniment to a meal, creating a complex interplay of tastes that stimulates the mind and offering a much more satisfying experience; it also elevates the meal's ritual value, helping you to see eating in a different light. Wine lends an atmosphere of seriousness, conviviality, refinement, and luxury, all of which counter the tendency to eat mindlessly and disrespectfully. (If you've opened a bottle of wine, you're not likely to eat in front of the television!)

Wine can also enhance your health if absorbed in small daily doses and always, always, *always* with food. (French women find it utterly odd to sit sipping a glass of Chardonnay as if it were a cocktail. The full taste of wine reveals itself only when paired with the right food.) Aside from containing fewer calories per volume than most alcoholic drinks, fine wine is also full of nutrients and recognized to thin the blood and lower blood pressure and bad cholesterol. How many undiluted pleasures can make such claims?

For Americans, the trouble seems to be either intimidation—"Which wine should I pick?"—or false assumptions—"Wine?

Oh sure, we have some on special occasions." For French people, wine is a part of everyday life, and most don't fuss too much over the choices. Most French people, in fact, know only about the wines of the region they live in. Nevertheless, I believe it is an important reason why French women don't get fat.

Introducing children to wine is pretty typical in France. We see our parents drink a glass with each meal, and naturally we want to taste. We were usually offered a little bit mixed with water at Sunday lunch. Sometimes, though, mischief will win out. I remember some pretty long meals with extended family—after a cousin's first communion, for instance—when some of the kids, mainly the boys, would wait until the grown-ups had got up to stretch in the garden. That was the cue to steal into the empty dining room and attack the glasses and bottles that weren't entirely empty. There was Champagne, white, red, dessert wine—all of it swirled together and passed around, as fast as the little scavengers could manage. Usually, the drinking party didn't last very long. But it was long enough: by the time they got caught, they were already sick, some parting with their lunch. Still, it was another lesson that can't be learned too early: "Drink in moderation, and don't mix!"

My first official introduction to wine—it is not apocryphal—actually happened in the heart of bubblyland, an hour or so from where I grew up in Lorraine. There lived two of my parents' best friends: a bon vivant architect working for the city of Reims, the Champagne capital of the world, and his tiny, adorable wife. She, alas, was not such a great cook and depended on her husband as her gastronomic savior, calling him *mon petit Jésus.* He, like my father, was a member of the pigeon society. The Lions would come often for my mother's celebrated *déjeuner du dimanche,* when Monsieur Lion would lend his own genius to the effort, concocting with my mother ever more fabulous meals. To reciprocate the hospitality, they would invite us and other friends to Reims, where M. Lion would let my mother take the lead in his wonderful kitchen. She had two kitchens to choose from. On their large estate, they had a main house and a summer cottage. The summer house kitchen was all white tile with state-of-the-art equipment; the winter house kitchen was like a museum, with wonderful antique ceramic ovens and decor. *Mamie* loved it, and everyone was gaga over her cooking.

A few times a year, we would leave home early Sunday morning, and my mother, given carte blanche, would cook all morning *chez Lion.* When the guests arrived, Champagne was served, and M. Lion felt that children should have *une petite goutte* (a tiny sip). I'll never forget it. First he taught us how to hold the glass. It was not the water tumbler from which we kids tasted our wine cut with water back home. That was not the right vessel for the king of wines! M. Lion meant to initiate me into one of the world's great rituals. Imagine a six-year-old holding a Champagne flute: with my pudgy little hand grasping the bowl, M. Lion explained this would warm the Champagne. He showed me the correct way to hold the tulip-shaped glass, by the stem or the foot. I was impressed. M. Lion was a huge man by French standards, and he had that puzzling nickname, so up until that moment I had found him rather intimidating. Now, I had the little Jesus as my friend. And he loved Champagne. Such delightful confusion. I still remember my first thrilling sips with the grown-up glass. For once, I had a great weekend story to share with my classmates on Monday. None of them had ever tried Champagne, much less held a proper Champagne glass! It made up for all the weekends I'd been dragged mushroom picking—not very cool for French kids—while my pals went to the movies. (My family insisted time together had to be about food, not sitting silently in the dark watching a film.)

It turns out that the Champagne I drank was Veuve Clicquot. And a few months later, on one of our regular visits to the Lions, we were taken to the property of the famous Champagne house. It was their favorite, and when we were ready to depart late on Sunday, M. Lion would load a case into our trunk as a thank-you to my mother. So it became our favorite, too. Not surprising: quality is never a hard sell. But little did I know that the grand name of Veuve Clicquot would become my life's work.

When I was a student in Paris, after I'd trimmed down with the help of Dr. Miracle, I decided to have a party to celebrate the end of term. I blithely went to the store to collect six bottles of Champagne. To my shock, and the proprietor's amusement, I had barely enough money for one! When I told my mother the story during our regular Sunday phone call, she took pity on me and volunteered to send me a check. She had taught us the value of most things, but unfortunately not the price. That was an adult lesson.

All my university friends were duly impressed. My precious offering was figuratively and literally the toast of the class. Champagne never fails to set a mood. Its festivity is irrepressible. Having learned this, I decided right there that, henceforth, I would either save up to have a party with Champagne or have no party at all. It makes all the difference.

I am truly one of those lucky people who get paid to do something they enjoy. You see, I still get a kick from Champagne—a big one. To me Champagne is magic. It's also a supremely feminine wine. I love everything about it: the seductive honey color, the tiny bubbles (they should dance for you), the scents and tastes (citrus, pear, apple, dried fruit, brioche), the lovely, long, yeasty aftertaste. I love the mood Champagne creates, the feeling no other wine can come close to: celebration, life-affirming joy. I find Champagne a most forgiving wine, too. The drama in the glass makes it hard to drink it too quickly, and I've never been drunk from it or had a Champagne hangover. Of course, I drink it in moderation and always with food. As with all good things in life, balance is the word.

For more than twenty centuries, the wines of Champagne have been present at happy occasions all over the world, but only since the Industrial Revolution in the late eighteenth century have we commoners had access to it. Before then, it was the wine of kings and the upper crust.

For the last few decades, I have been spoiled by the chance to share an almost daily glass of Champagne with someone my work has allowed me to know, whether in Paris, New York, Santa Barbara, Bali, Sardinia, Kyoto, Mykonos, Provence, Puerto Rico, San Francisco, Miami, Nantucket, or countless other places. As Edward tells me, "You make people happy. It's like having a magic wand!"

I have always known this. When I first moved to New York, I had to visit a friend in the hospital. Naturally, I brought a bottle of Champagne. French custom calls for bringing either Champagne or flowers, and knowing my friend, I opted for the former. But the duty nurse wouldn't even let me through the door. It was a startling moment of culture clash. In America, with its history of temperance movements and the Eighteenth Amendment, Champagne in a hospital seems scandalous. In France, you'll often see cartoons of a doctor sitting by a convalescent's bedside, drinking to the patient's health.

Today when I lunch with friends, I find we are often the only people in the restaurant drinking Champagne, even if our food is a simple platter of oysters with some great bread and butter. What could they be "celebrating" at noon? the people sipping bright orange cocktails at the bar seem to wonder. Life, I suppose. Marlene Dietrich used to say Champagne gives the impression that every day is Sunday. That sums it up well.

In France today, Champagne bars are popping up all over. The variety is wonderful. In fact, though, one of the longest-running Champagne bars is in Chicago, Pop's for Champagne, where I've been going for more than twenty years.

Champagne remains my best trick to whet my appetite and awaken my palate. (Remember, being ready for the pleasure of food is essential to contentment with proper proportion.) It's also a wine that can accompany a meal, complementing so many foods—did you know it pairs perfectly with pizza, the acidity contrasting with the oil and cheese? I wouldn't go so far as some who say it goes with everything, but it is unquestionably the most versatile wine there is. You can get fancy with different vintages and even serve rosé. Or you can simply enjoy that year's brut for roughly the price of a good bottle of still wine. Just keep it simple: avoid serving Champagne with sauces that are very spicy or heavy with cream. Also don't pair it with the few foods that neutralize its flavors: artichokes, asparagus, and chocolate. Cooking with Champagne is also fun. It's much more elegant than using a simple white wine, and as you'll need only a little, you can have the rest of the bottle with the meal.

Here's a perfect recipe for dinner *à deux*, bound to impress your date. When I serve it to guests they always ask for the recipe and think I've been cooking for hours, but it is done in little more than half an hour. And there is zero fat added; the chicken cooks in Champagne. Cooking with wine adds flavor, but the calories of the alcohol burn off in the pan. Vermouth, Pernod, or any number of earthy reds or whites can add depth to a dish, but for elegance of finish nothing beats Champagne. I often make this dish on a workday when pressed for time, especially when entertaining on a weeknight. Once you get it going, it needs no minding, giving you ample time to prepare the rest of the dinner. The recipe makes enough for four, so I have the leftovers to make some nice chicken sandwiches.

CHICKEN AU CHAMPAGNE
Serves 4

Start with the best and most flavorful fresh chicken you can find. Organic, free-range chicken is more widely available than ever. As for the Champagne, I recommend Veuve Clicquot Yellow Label Brut. (Quelle surprise!) Okay, here's my disclaimer: I work for the company, but I am also addicted to its rich, full-bodied style and quality. Lots of good sparkling wines are made around the world, but they don't taste the same as French Champagne. And even Champagnes vary a good deal, depending on the grapes used, winemaking, and aging. Champagne has two reliable properties for cooking (or drinking). The first is dryness. Champagne is an austere wine, high in acidity. With chicken, I am not looking for sweetness, so Brut is the style of Champagne that works best. Second, I consider the flavors the wine imparts to the chicken. Veuve Clicquot is notable for its rich, full body and full flavor, having been made mostly from red grapes (Pinot Noir and Pinot Meunier) with about a third Chardonnay.

INGREDIENTS

4 chicken breasts (with skin and bone)

Salt and freshly ground pepper

Chervil, tarragon, or thyme (optional)

1 shallot, quartered

1 cup Champagne (Veuve Clicquot Yellow Label Brut recommended)

1. Place the chicken breasts in a roasting pan, and season them. Pour ½ cup of the Champagne over breasts. Make a slit in each breast and insert a piece of shallot.

2. Place the pan under the broiler, skin-side down, for 3 minutes, until the skin is nicely browned. Turn and broil the other side for 5 minutes.

3. Remove the chicken from the broiler, baste with the pan juices, and add the remaining ½ cup of Champagne. Adjust the oven

temperature to 475 degrees and bake the chicken for 30 minutes, basting once or twice.

4. Serve over brown rice. Sautéed mushrooms add a special touch and go beautifully with Champagne. (In a warm frying pan with a touch of olive oil, add clean, roughly chopped mushrooms, and cook for a few minutes. Add a few drops of lemon juice, freshly chopped sage, seasoning to taste, and 1 tablespoon of butter.) Pour the cooking juices from the chicken over the meat and rice. Serve the remainder of the bottle of Champagne (about 6 glasses) with the meal.

While Champagne is my first choice in wine, when it's not available or appropriate, I enjoy a glass of anything good to great (which doesn't, by any means, equal expensive) and have white or red favorites from just about everywhere in the world where wine is produced. I like dry whites, love a good Chablis, Meursault, or a dry Riesling from my beloved Alsace, a Sauvignon Blanc from New Zealand, or an unfiltered Chardonnay from the Napa Valley. As for reds, I opt for the round, soft, light to medium types, such as a Volnay from Burgundy and other Pinot Noirs, or reds from Tuscany or, for something bigger, the Rhône. I am not really a fan of those big, tannic, high-alcohol Cabernets, although some foods ask for a big one, and I love to answer.

As I get older, I find sticking to one or two grape varietals throughout a meal—as opposed to switching from course to course to various wines blended from different grapes—is easier on my body. And I never touch spirits. In wine you must learn your preferences and be ready to adjust them over time. My first choices are Chardonnay and Pinot Noir. Getting to know a few different grapes is a good way to start your appreciation of wine. Here is not the place for a discourse on food and wine pairings, but to illustrate my point about some classic marriages that are richly rewarding, I offer the following examples to get you thinking: Pinot Noir with salmon or duck; Cabernet Sauvignon with steak and grilled meats; Zinfandel with turkey; Chardonnay with chicken or lobster; Sauvignon Blanc with shrimp; Champagne with just about anything. In sum, there are two rules for pairing food and wine that I live by. Rule one: Have red wine with meat; white wine with fish and poultry. Rule two: Forget rule one and please yourself by pairing any food with any wine as long as you write the individual formula that works for you and yields the most pleasure at the table.

Now, how much of a good thing is the right amount for you? On average, women just can't drink as much as men, but I find a glass or two a day does more than any apple to keep the doctor away. Besides, I can't really enjoy lunch or dinner without a glass of wine.

Still, we all face the temptation to overdo it from time to time: long meals in restaurants, holiday gatherings, or other festive occasions when it seems the glass is always kept full. As I have described, my own work puts me in temptation's way constantly, and too much alcohol not only loosens inhibitions (a potential professional disaster), but also encourages overeating (an equilibrium buster).

I learned a valuable trick early in my career. When I first entered the wine business, I was a guest at a large Champagne house where day in and day out some twenty to thirty people were guests for lunch and dinner. There was both a full-time staff and a full-time hostess (and PR lady), a wonderful countess in her late forties.

One day, we were served six wines with a lunch that lasted well over three hours. Some guests left the table noticeably looped. But the countess got up as fresh as a rose and, catching my admiring look, took me to one side, pleased to share her simple trick: At any meal, she would limit her total intake to one glass simply by *pretending* to drink most of the time. She recommended I watch her that night at dinner. As hostess, she'd be the one to speak, whether in welcome or to raise a toast, so she was naturally the center of attention. What nobody noticed was that she'd barely put her lips to the glass and then swallow only a drop or two. When the waiter came around with the wine, her glass was still filled, so he'd skip her and refill the glasses of the others, none of whom noticed. Some guests would have had two or three glasses when the countess had barely drunk a third of her glass. This she repeated over the remaining courses, assuring she didn't down more than a glass in total, but never appearing less than the picture of conviviality. Without applying the countess's secret daily, I'd never have managed to hold on to my job all these years, since like her, I must frequently entertain at lunch and dinner. As she knew very well, when you are promoting the pleasures of food and drink, your dinner guests must never suspect you've had a three-course meal with wine at lunch.

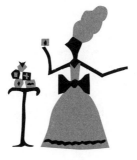

9

BREAD AND CHOCOLATE

I recently saw a short play in Paris called *Les Mangeuses de Chocolat* (loosely translated, *Women Who Eat Chocolate*). Three young addicts decide to try group therapy, and the therapist (an ex-chocoholic herself) will try to help each find her *élément déclencheur* (key to getting unhooked). They all fail (surprise), and nothing gets resolved (this is French theater), but there are lots of good lines, some with more than a grain of truth. For instance: A survey reveals that nine out of ten people admit to loving chocolate . . . and the tenth one is lying.

The play was satirizing a French obsession (chocolate), but also the therapeutic establishment, which perhaps one couldn't get away with in America. I took it in good fun, except when a comment was made about women who eat their chocolate *en cachette* (in private). To the French, the idea seems silly enough for a gag, but given my American experience, I couldn't laugh. Too often, American women eat on the sly, and the result is much more guilt than pleasure. The tendency goes with an attitude that should be changed. Nothing is *sinfully* delicious. If you really enjoy something, as I adore chocolate, there is a place for it in your life. But we cannot allow guilt-ridden scarfing. Only with cultivated pleasure can you enjoy chocolate in the clear light of day. The same goes for other excellent foods Americans have come to consider no-no's.

French women eat chocolate (about twelve pounds a year on average). They also eat bread (we fought a revolution over it!), another item on our watch list of offenders. But: *French women don't get fat.* In fact, here's another form of the French Paradox: Pretending such pleasures don't exist, or trying to eliminate them from your diet for an extended time, will probably lead to weight gain. The only long-term effect of deprivation is the yo-yo—down today, but up again before you know it. It's utterly pointless, especially because both bread and chocolate are good for you.

If we are going to eat bread and chocolate (and we are) and not get fat (and we are not), we need to use our heads, as Dr. Miracle advised. Maximize the rewards of pleasure while minimizing the costs. In fact, he insisted little pleasures (*menus plaisirs*) were the key to success, and according to his prescription, I absolutely needed to have my chocolate, but in little doses (*par petites doses*). I also had to cultivate my appreciation for what I was having. In short, he taught me the French way of enjoying those foods that can be friend or foe depending on how we treat them. The keys are sensory awareness, portion sense, quality, and an eye to the big picture of overall wellness (*bien-être*).

I've already confessed that *je raffole de chocolat,* which basically means I am a chocoholic. I'm convinced I inherited that gene from my mother. She had an amazing repertoire of chocolate desserts, as well as a passion for straight consumption. It made her the easiest person in the world to shop for. Bringing back chocolate from Belgium, Switzerland, or any good French chocolatier was a sure way to her heart. Some years ago, when a famous chocolatier in Lyon passed away in his late seventies, the obituary in *Le Monde* revealed he had eaten one *tablette* (a good-size chocolate bar) a day for most of his life. The joke in our family became that there was now proof of at least one person in France who had eaten more chocolate than my mother. But since she would live past ninety, enjoying chocolate all her days, I'm sure she beat him out in the end.

If the magnitude of the chocolatier's habit doesn't sound impressive to you, your relation to chocolate must be examined. For the man from Lyon was, by French standards, extraordinary—few of us could eat as much and still eat it properly. Not that enjoying chocolate is a competitive sport. In fact, when Mother was enjoying her fix, it was more like Zen meditation. No one talked. One look at her expressions, her lips, her eyes, commanded a hush in the house. It was a natural way of honoring our mother, allowing her the moment to savor one of her most elemental pleasures. To know how to appreciate that burst of delicate flavors, that supreme smoothness of texture as it melts in your mouth and begins its way down your throat, is to me a great accomplishment of sensual eating. It's an experience that could not be more remote from eating a Snickers bar on the run. But how did this gentle madness evolve? History reveals there are deep roots to the allure of *Theobroma cacao,* the technical term for chocolate, meaning in Greek "food of the gods."

Chocolate came to Europe via the New World, in the age of more than one discovery. The Olmecs (1500–600 B.C.) seem to have happened on it first. Their idea of chocolate was as a high-energy drink, extremely bitter and peppery, and a sort of proto–PowerBar reserved for men (priests, princes, and warriors); they believed the magic food would improve war making, sexual prowess, and one's chances of surviving snakebite. But our own version may be traced to the later pre-Columbian civilizations, around 3000 B.C., when wild cacao trees grew in the warm and humid soils of Mesoamerica, modern-day Mexico and Guatemala.

For the Aztecs and Totecs, chocolate was not only an elixir, but a symbol of value. Their system of commerce was based on the cocoa standard, and the chocolate produced was consumed by noblemen and merchants (all men, of course) at banquets. It was still very bitter and peppery, but it was mixed with vanilla, honey, and flowers and served cold and foamy, usually at the end of a meal along with the tubes for smoking tobacco. Apart from its energizing powers (these blends were highly caffeinated, no doubt), it was believed to be an aphrodisiac. The emperor Montezuma is known to have consumed huge quantities, of various colors in golden cups, before paying a visit to his harem!

Europeans first tried chocolate following the fourth voyage of Columbus in 1502, but the Spanish appear to have been unimpressed until 1528, when Cortez brought back not only cocoa beans, but a recipe and tools for making chocolate. It became a Spanish sensation. After that, the direction of global conquest was reversed, at least gastronomically. Europe has remained a continent of chocolate fanatics ever since. Louis XIV's wife, Marie-Thérèse, is reported to have assured the Sun King that she had no passions except for her husband and chocolate (although one wonders which she valued more). By the nineteenth century, no less an authority than history's greatest gastronome, Brillat-Savarin, proclaimed, "Chocolate is health," and he prescribed it for many ills long before science confirmed its therapeutic properties.

In its pure dark form, chocolate has indeed been shown to be "heart smart," with more antioxidants than black tea or red wine, as well as lots of magnesium, iron, and potassium (all vital to women's health). It can also ease anxiety and depression, as it contains serotonin and theobromine, which act on brain receptors and have a beneficial influence on mood. As it is also high in fat, however, it is better enjoyed after lighter meals than after fat-laden holiday feasts, or by itself as a pick-me-up.

One of the most dispiriting developments of the twentieth century was the mass production of chocolate. It created an inferior product loaded with bad fats, and as a result, many Americans have never in their lives tasted the real thing. But relief has appeared with the rise of new artisanal chocolatiers, passionate guardians of traditional methods that were perfected in the eighteenth century. It is to these chocolate makers, now popping up across America, that we must look for the quality that first inspired chocolate worship. My mantra of quality over quantity is doubly important when applied to something as potent as chocolate.

Quality chocolate is labor-intensive and complex. It requires careful orchard selection, cultivation, and then harvest of the precious fruit. Next comes fermentation and two rounds of drying, followed by roasting and a few more delicate procedures before one obtains the cocoa mass. The proof of adequate attention and skill will be in the pudding, literally. From that mass, three products are extracted: liquor, cocoa butter, and cocoa powder. These are the materials from which the artisan works, making chocolate slabs, ganache (a mixture of chocolate with either butter, crème fraîche, or a milk product), *praliné* (a mixture of sugar and ground almonds or hazelnuts with chocolate), or chocolate filled with fruit or liquor. Toto, I don't think we're in Hershey, Pennsylvania, anymore.

In tasting chocolate, sweetness, saltiness, acidity, and bitterness are key savors. Acidity is what you should feel inside your cheeks, and it's essential to the diffusion of aromas and length of taste in the mouth. Bitterness is felt at the tip of the tongue. It signals a chocolate with little sugar, and it's a good quality as long as it does not cancel out any other sensation. Texture is also vitally important to character: smoothness, the crunch of the shell. The artisan's ability to play with the yin and yang of chocolate—sweet-salty, sweet-bitter, acid-bitter, hard-soft, crispy-luscious, cold-warm—explains why the experience of one master's work can differ meaningfully from the experience of another's work.

For French women, the real thing remains dark chocolate, bittersweet or, even better, extra-bittersweet, which is the purest, with the highest percentage of cocoa solids—the stuff that makes chocolate taste chocolatey. Although you rarely meet someone who "doesn't like chocolate," what the average American consumes, a chocolate connoisseur would never touch: milk chocolate, white chocolate, or any of the various packaged forms sold in supermarkets and drugstores. This is, quite simply, junk food, loaded with sugar, very low in cocoa content, and more often than not artificially colored and preserved (real chocolate, like fresh-ground coffee, has a very short life of full flavor).

Admittedly, we French get carried away with chocolate: we have chocolate museums and clubs. We have magazines dedicated to chocolate, a *université du chocolat,* and *salons du chocolat* (fairs). There are tastings and competitions for the best chocolate soufflé, the finest chocolate macaroon. Some Parisians will cross the Seine simply to buy the *grains de café* (chocolate in the shape of coffee beans) from a particular shop. And France being France, there is *une Académie du chocolat,* for ultimate authority. Whenever I would come home with a good report card, my mother would say, *"Tu mérites la médaille en chocolat"* ("You've earned the chocolate medal"). It was a bittersweet compliment: in a country where national honors are routinely doled out according to connections, only a distinction of chocolate could be an honest acknowledgment of merit.

The value of good chocolate holds steady. Many French women say, *"Je déprime donc je chocolate"* ("When I'm down, I chocolate," meaning, I splurge on the dark stuff). When you come to recognize the potential for taste pleasure and psychic relief, you will understand that it's worth the investment. Fortunately, with good chocolate you don't need—and should not want—pounds of it for pleasure. A couple of choice pieces a day won't disable your budget or your weight-maintenance program. For those not near the chocolate boutiques now appearing in most American cities, it is possible to order high quality online, such as dark, rich, delicious Valrhona.

And of course, using a little "food of the gods" can elevate the simplest dessert to a sacrament.

Here are four of my favorite family recipes embracing chocolate.

CHOCOLATE RICE PUDDING

Serves 4

This perfect comfort food is a wonderful winter dessert that's easy and quick to make before your guests arrive and leave on the counter till dessert time.

INGREDIENTS

2 cups milk

½ cup sugar

Pinch of salt

1 cup arborio rice

½ teaspoon pure vanilla extract

3 ounces dark chocolate (80 percent cacao preferred), broken into small pieces

1. Pour the milk, sugar, and pinch of salt into a saucepan and bring to a boil over low heat. Add the rice and cook for 20 minutes, stirring occasionally, until the milk is absorbed (if the mixture becomes sticky, add a bit more milk to keep the rice creamy). Stir in the vanilla.

2. Pour the rice pudding into 4 ramekins and using a spoon, insert the chocolate pieces in the middle of each mold and push them into the rice. Leave at room temperature. The chocolate will slowly melt and mix with the pudding. Let your guests play with the way they want to eat it: mix the whole thing together or start by eating the rice laced with melted chocolate and the chocolate center separately—a matter of taste and mood and a tough decision.

CHOCOLATE-ESPRESSO FAUX SOUFFLÉS

Serves 4

Soufflés are easy to make once you know the technique and have had some practice, but they are not practical to make when entertaining, as they require your attention and time away from your guests. Plus, the fear of the soufflé falling is not worth the risk. Instead, here's a recipe you can prepare ahead of time for a cold soufflé that is yummy and impressive.

INGREDIENTS

8 ounces dark chocolate (over 70 percent cacao minimum)

4 egg whites

Salt

4 egg yolks

2 tablespoons strong espresso coffee

1. Melt the chocolate in the top of a double boiler set over a pan of simmering water on medium heat.

2. Beat the egg whites with a pinch of salt until stiff, glossy white peaks are formed.

3. Whisk the egg yolks into the chocolate. Stir in the coffee. Gently fold in ⅓ of the whites, and then fold in the rest.

4. Pour the soufflé mixture into 4 molds, cover with plastic wrap, and refrigerate for 4 hours before serving.

N.B. THOUGH MOST AMERICANS APPROACH RAW EGGS WITH MORE TREPIDATION THAN IS, PERHAPS, NECESSARY, IT IS BEST NOT TO SERVE DISHES INCORPORATING UNCOOKED EGGS TO PREGNANT WOMEN, SMALL CHILDREN, SENIORS, AND PEOPLE WITH IMMUNE-SYSTEM DEFICIENCIES. AND ORGANIC EGGS FROM FREE-RANGE CHICKENS ARE ALWAYS THE SAFEST—TASTIEST, TOO.

MOUSSE AU CHOCOLAT

Serves 6 (¹/₂ cup per person)

There are at least a dozen chocolate mousse recipes in my family. (Most French families have multiple preparations for this dessert, which is the preeminent standard and choice for homemade chocolate desserts.) All of them are good, but this one is a favorite for its purity (no butter, no coffee, very little sugar, and more egg whites than yolks, which makes for an airy mousse, the perfect dessert after a rich meal).

1. Melt the chocolate in the top of a double boiler set over a pan of simmering water on medium heat.

2. Remove the chocolate from the heat and add the sugar. Stir well and add the egg yolks, one at a time.

3. Beat the egg whites until stiff, glossy peaks are formed. Gently fold the whites into the chocolate mixture until well blended.

4. Pour the mousse into a serving bowl, cover with plastic wrap, and refrigerate overnight.

INGREDIENTS

4 ounces dark chocolate (80 percent cacao preferred)

1 tablespoon sugar

3 egg yolks

5 egg whites

TARTINE AU CACAO

Serves 1

This "kid's food" works as a dessert, snack, or dinner. Following a full and balanced lunch, our nanny loved those evenings when she could feed us this easy tartine and leave once we were done. Her only complaint was that she always had to wipe my face, barbouillée de cacao *(smeared with chocolate), and she had to clean me up before joining her boyfriend, who was waiting for her outside. The kid in me continues to splurge occasionally on this evening tartine.*

INGREDIENTS

1 ounce crème fraîche (sour cream is a close approximation, and good-quality cream cheese works, too)

1 thick slice of country bread (sourdough is good, too)

1 tablespoon cocoa powder

1. Spread a thick layer of crème fraîche on the bread and dust with the cocoa powder.

2. Serve with ½ cup of homemade hot chocolate.

. . . .

Finally, a little pool of melted chocolate is an irresistible setting for a piece of poached fruit and can bump a simple dessert up one level in luxury.

I was recently seated next to a famous New York restaurateur, who said to me, "Isn't it terrible that no one in New York eats bread anymore?" Since the carb police have been patrolling twenty-four hours a day, bread seems to have become public enemy number one. To me it's just sad that so many people are forgoing one of life's most elemental pleasures for the sake of a dead-end weight-loss strategy. It's sadder still that the adherents of the strategy would rather risk heart disease than let a bit of bread pass their lips. Does bread make people fat? Ridiculous! Too much of most things will make you fat, of course. But there's nothing wrong with bread per se. Eliminating it from one's diet is lamentable, probably unhealthy . . . and very un-French. The French say, *"On ne badine pas avec l'amour"* ("You don't fool around with love"). To us, the same goes for bread, an old flame we will never part with.

Don't get me wrong. I don't insist bread has to be in your life. Hundreds of millions of people on this planet get on fine without it. But if you appreciate good bread, as I do, be advised that you can enjoy it while still managing a healthy weight.

Good bread is rich in fiber and vital for *le transit intestinal,* and we French care about our digestion as much as our alimentation. And since French bread contains no fat and tends toward lightness, it's not the sort of calorie pack you need to approach all that cautiously. But French women do have their ground rules about it. We count our slices and do not eat bread before our first course is served, avoiding a great pitfall of dining out: the bread pre-appetizer. It's a simple trick worth learning. Unless you are faint from hunger, you can hold out for ten minutes and save a good number of calories and room for your balanced meal.

A slice or two of bread *with* a meal (or as a meal) is one of our great pleasures. One slice (about an inch thick if it's the silver-dollar baguette diameter) has no more calories than a piece of fruit and, being a starch, releases sugar more slowly. With a little something extra (a couple of sardines, a slice of truffle, what-have-you) and some butter, it can be a wonderfully satisfying, balanced little meal unto itself. *Tartine beurrée* (bread and butter) is great for breakfast; *jambon-beurre* (ham on a buttered baguette), the classic French sandwich, makes a popular lunch. In American sandwiches, the bread seems incidental; in French sandwiches, it's the filling that offers the occasion to eat bread. Not that you need an occasion. My mother would regularly break off a piece of baguette at around eleven a.m. and eat it as a *coupe faim*.

The biggest obstacle for Americans is not the amount of the bread they consume, but the quality. In this respect, alas, they are not alone. Most European countries have lost the traditional knack for good bread. Even in Italy, where food reaches heights to rival those in France and is an equally serious affair, the quality of bread is not what it was. Italian friends who visit me in Paris are always in search of the best baguette and the best *pain au levain* or croissant (these last are subject to annual contests where I come from), which keeps France's great bakers on their toes.

They have to be, because the French simply do not tolerate bad bread. I have seen Parisian friends complain about the bread to the owners of a little neighborhood bistro with otherwise delicious food. Granted, it was not the best bread I ever had, but it was hardly the inedible industrial kind one might get in a somewhat comparable New York restaurant. No matter; by the next visit, I noticed they had changed bakers. Can you imagine that in any other country?

We share a set of standards and expectations. The baguette has to be *croustillante* (crispy and crusty), with large, irregular air holes, while we look for *moelleux* (softness and unctuousness) and acidity in the white of the *pain au levain*. And there are food assignments. With oysters we like *pain de seigle* (a light brown bread that's two-thirds rye and one-third wheat flour). With our cheese we love walnut or hazelnut bread, not just any nut bread, and, of course, olive bread has become a staple not just in Provence, but as an accompaniment to Mediterranean fare anywhere, particularly fish preparations. Still, bread is never reduced to the ordinary, and as with other things, we take pleasure in exploring all its sensual possibilities.

I would be misleading you, however, if I left the impression that France has been a paradise of bread during my whole life. In fact, from the 1960s through the 1980s, we endured a sort of national bread crisis—what we French ironically call "the industrial ersatz period," when time-honored methods and tools were replaced by industrial equipment and techniques. It was a Gaullist idea of progress, I suppose. Fortunately, that is mostly behind us, though remnants of that age can still be found in plastic bags in the *hypermarchés*. Thanks to an American named Steven Kaplan, a professor at Cornell University as well as a Francophile and bread lover, and to the former prime minister Edouard Balladur, reform legislation was passed in 1993. The now famous Balladur Law has immensely improved, or rather reclaimed, the traditional standards for French bread. Regulating flour quality, yeast content, fermentation techniques, and taste, it has made certain that no French-bread lover will ever again be left behind. Today, tradition is safely entrusted to a new generation of devoted artisanal bakers. They take pride not only in getting it right, but in making it better, recognizing that the reputation of the nation is at stake.

To my great satisfaction, these new bakers have their spiritual confrères in America. The bread renaissance is a vital part of the American artisanal movement, and there has been a proliferation of specialty shops and new offerings in the farmers' markets, as I find at my favorite haunt, New York's Union Square.

But if you don't live near a devoted artisan—and it's hit or miss outside major cities—what's an American woman to do without access to great bread? When I first moved to New York, I was in that very boat. It forced me to do something few French women ever need to do: learn to bake my own. What was even tougher, I had to learn to make croissants to answer a hardwired Sunday morning craving that simply would not respond to Sara Lee or the greasy abominations chain bakeries call croissants.

For those who may consider baking bread as much a backward waste of time as taking your laundry down to the river, I offer the wisdom of the great American gastronome M.F.K. Fisher, who in *The Art of Eating* wrote, "No yoga exercise, no meditation in a chapel filled with music will rid you of your blues better than the humble task of making your own bread." It's not that I can rival the bakers of Paris in quality. But nothing prepares one for the full experience of tasting great bread like the aromatic anticipation of baking it. And nothing equals the taste of bread in that first half hour out of the oven. Perhaps it's why in Paris, I time my weekends around the baking schedule of Carton, the great master in my neighborhood. Perhaps, too, it's why in New York, friends continue coming over on Sunday morning for my amateur croissants long after professional standards have improved. It's a willingness to reap the pleasures of food at its most elementally wonderful. French women don't eat Wonder Bread.

Try baking bread some weekend.

BAGUETTES

Makes 4

These 18- to 24-inch wands of French bread are as much a symbol of France as the Eiffel Tower. And while French women don't bake them today, when they are for sale on almost every commercial block of every town and city, there's no substitute for the intoxicating aromas of freshly baked bread at home. Good baguettes should be crusty, moist, slightly chewy, and, of course, flavorful. And they are amazingly easy to make. The water content depends on the flour and the weather.

INGREDIENTS

1 teaspoon active dry yeast

2 cups warm water

4 to 5 cups unbleached all-purpose white flour

2 teaspoons kosher salt

1 egg, beaten and mixed with 1 tablespoon cold water

1. In a small bowl dissolve yeast in ½ cup warm water. Stir with a fork. Set aside for 10 minutes.

2. Combine the flour and salt. Add the yeast mixture, and stir in the remaining 1½ cups water. Mix the dough until it is sticky enough to knead. On a lightly floured board, knead for 6 to 10 minutes; the dough should be sticky and smooth. Put the dough in a bowl, cover with a damp tea towel, and let rise at room temperature until doubled in volume, about one hour.

3. Punch down the dough and divide into 4 pieces. Roll each into a ball and shape into a baguette. Transfer the loaves to a lightly greased baking sheet (I use a special baguette-shaped baking pan) and let rise until nearly doubled.

4. Preheat the oven to 450 degrees. Brush the baguettes with the egg-water mixture. Score the loaves diagonally across the top with a sharp knife.

5. Pour 2 cups of hot water into a pan and place in the preheated oven next to the baguettes to provide moisture. Bake the baguettes for 15 minutes, and then lower the temperature to 400 degrees and bake for 5 to 10 minutes more, until golden brown. Remove from the oven and cool on a rack before slicing.

CROISSANTS

Makes 12

Croissants are created in stages; it takes time to "grow" them. You will need to start on Friday to enjoy your Sunday a.m. epiphany, but the individual steps are rather quick and in all take only about 1½ hours. And the technique is not difficult to master; after a few times you'll be an expert croissant baker.

INGREDIENTS

1 cup milk plus 2 tablespoons to brush over croissants

2 teaspoons active dry yeast

2¼ cups plus 3 tablespoons sifted all-purpose flour (measure and reserve in separate bowls)

2 tablespoons sugar

1 teaspoon salt

12 tablespoons sweet (unsalted) butter

FOR GLAZE:

1 egg yolk mixed with 1 tablespoon milk

FRIDAY EVENING (DAY 1):

1. Heat 1 cup of the milk to lukewarm. Dissolve the yeast in ¼ cup of the lukewarm milk. Stir in 2 tablespoons flour (from the 2¼ cups) and whisk until there are no lumps. Cover with plastic wrap and let stand at room temperature until doubled in volume (this will take about 20 minutes).

2. Mix the sugar and salt into the 2⅛ cups flour.

3. Heat the remaining milk. Transfer the raised dough to the bowl of an electric mixer fitted with the dough hook, add the lukewarm milk, and with the mixer at high speed, start adding the sugar, salt, and flour (from step 2), a little at a time, reducing the speed to low-medium until the dough is sticky and soft.

4. Cover the bowl with plastic wrap and refrigerate overnight.

1. Bring the butter to room temperature and work it with the heel of your hand to incorporate the remaining 3 tablespoons of flour until smooth. Shape into a square.

2. Sprinkle the work surface (a marble slab is ideal) with the flour, shape the cold dough into a 6 × 15-inch rectangle, and spread the butter square on the upper ⅔ of the rectangle, leaving a ½-inch border around the sides and top. Fold the dough like a letter into thirds. Turn the dough counterclockwise (it will look like a notebook with the open flap on your right), and then again roll out the dough into a 6 × 15-inch rectangle and fold as before.

3. Transfer the dough to a baking pan, cover with plastic wrap, and refrigerate for 6 hours.

Roll out the dough 2 more times, wrap, and refrigerate overnight.

1. About 1½ hours before baking time, remove the dough from the refrigerator and sprinkle flour on the work surface. Roll the dough into a 16-inch circle, working as quickly as possible. Using a knife, cut the dough into quarters and then cut each quarter into 3 triangles.

2. With both hands, roll the base of each triangle toward the remaining corner. Do not curl the ends in a croissant shape. Transfer the croissants to a baking sheet and brush with 2 tablespoons

milk. Let stand at room temperature for about 45 minutes, or until the croissants have doubled in volume.

3. Preheat the oven to 400 degrees. Brush the croissants with the glaze and bake for 15 to 20 minutes. If the croissants brown too fast, cover them loosely with foil and continue baking. Let cool 20 minutes before serving.

. . . .

POPPY SEED ROLLS

Makes 12

Amazingly, neither my mother nor my tante *Berthe ever used a recipe or a cookbook, and although this recipe (adapted from what I remembered watching) is good, I confess I have never tasted the equal of* Tante *Berthe's delicious rolls. Replacing poppy seeds with cumin yields one more recipe variation from Alsace.*

INGREDIENTS

1. Mix together the egg and water. Reserve.

2. Whip the yogurt and olive oil to a smooth consistency. Sift together the flour, sugar, salt, and baking powder. Make a well and pour the yogurt-oil mixture into the center. Using your fingertips, mix the dough until it is homogeneous. Work the dough until it no longer sticks and has a smooth consistency.

3. Preheat the oven to 400 degrees. Make 12 round rolls and put on a baking sheet. Brush with the egg-water mixture and sprinkle with poppy seeds. Using a sharp knife, make a cross on top of each roll. Bake in the preheated oven for 30 minutes, or until the rolls are golden. They are good warm, but you can, of course, serve them at room temperature once cooled.

1 egg

1 tablespoon water

1⅓ cups plain yogurt (page 151, or if you buy it make sure it's unsweetened and has no additives)

4 tablespoons olive oil

2½ cups unsifted all-purpose flour

2 tablespoons sugar

1 teaspoon salt

1 tablespoon double-acting baking powder

1 teaspoon poppy seeds

Although I don't like to dine late, by American standards I often do. Usually, it's eight or eight-thirty p.m. before I've been seated. In France, a true restaurant (as opposed to a bistro, brasserie, or a place that caters to tourists) won't even take a reservation before eight p.m., and most of the French don't arrive till nine. (Actually, that's nothing: in Spain and South America, they sit down at eleven p.m.) Nevertheless, having started the day by seven a.m., I'm always psychologically and physically in need of something before dinner. So it has taken some training to limit myself to a glass of Champagne or water and wait till food is served. I used to find myself immediately eating a slice or two of bread, at least in restaurants. As I have mentioned, I identified pre-dining bread as a problem well after my Dr. Miracle days. Recognizing an acquired offender (they can appear at any point) was important; cutting back was simple and produced results. Subtracting 12 or 15 unnecessary slices of bread per week will bless you with room for more conscious indulgences.

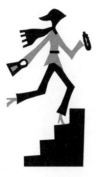

10

MOVING LIKE A FRENCH WOMAN

The great writer Colette was the first French woman to work out in the American sense. She would rise every morning and hit "the gym," a collection of primitive contraptions she even traveled with. To most French women, however, the idea holds little appeal. For while exerting oneself physically is completely essential to Montaigne's ideal of the healthy mind in a healthy body, dressing to break a sweat doesn't go with being French. Partly, it all seems such a great, joyless effort: cutting two hours out of the precious day—the travel, changing, learning to use machines, waiting to use them, showering, drying your hair, and so on. "And you have to pay for it!" as my friend Sylvie snickers. So while you will surely find all the latest apparatus in a good French hotel, know that they are there as a grudging concession to tourists and businesspeople. It's odd for a French woman to use them or to be seen jogging in the Luxembourg Gardens or the Tuileries.

Odd, but charming, too, because what French women do, they do out of their own desires. You see, we are all, to the core, *individualistes invétérées* (stubborn individualists), and as long as you are doing your own thing, it's fine. Some, though not many, French women enjoy sport: tennis and swimming are both fun and excellent for you. *Bon.* If your kick is running in the park, we say *amuse-toi bien* (have fun). It's only the view of the workout as mandatory sentence that rubs us the wrong way. It's the American rule of "No pain, no gain" that we reject.

A disproportionate amount of exercise, as some American women practice, may turn out to load the deck against your weight-loss goals. While offering little or no health benefit compared with milder exertion, the overheated workout may in fact lead to defeatism ("I give up!"), even to heartier eating. Indeed, too many women I know exercise so that they end up with oversize appetites just to refuel their bodies. They become like (gym) rats on a treadmill. It's obvious that someone is plotting against them: just look at all the offender foods stocked in gym cafés, awaiting these unsuspecting women after their two-hour session: sugary fruit juices, half-pound muffins, high-protein bars. You can cancel out your whole routine before you're even out the door! French women know any regimen you can't maintain for long stretches of life is bound to fail you, just as they know that boredom, not food, is the enemy.

American women seem to have two modes: sitting or

spinning. French women prefer the gentler, more regular varieties of all-day movement—"the slow burn," in American terms. And as you might expect, our approach, true to Cartesian principles, demands that you use your mind as you use your body. Mindless exercise is almost as bad as mindless eating. We strive to diversify the physical movement in our lives and practice it as second nature. And we cultivate awareness as we go.

French women see exertion as an integral part of the day. I encourage you to look at everyday movement, what you do in street clothes, as essential to your overall wellness and not to see exertion as something assigned to the gym. It may mean extra steps in the yard or not using interoffice mail. Or it may mean riding your bike to work or ironing your own clothes. The point is to practice as much physical exertion for as many moments of the day as you can manage. This is the surest way to overcome the mental hurdle that the idea of regular exercise presents to some of us. Reap the benefits without the bother. If you believe working at your desk leaves you no time for such things, you should realize that stress and fatigue in modern life typically have more to do with a lack of exertion than with too much.

À PIED

Here's a story about the Swiss you may not have heard. They are the world's biggest producers and consumers of chocolate—more than twenty pounds a year per person—yet they are not tipping the scales in the world weight-gaining Olympics. Why? Half of their run-of-the-mill getting around is done on foot or bicycle. Americans on average travel on their own steam less than 10 percent of the time. We French claim little resemblance to the Swiss except in the domains of chocolate and walking, where we are more than respectable performers.

Every time we are in France for a week or more, my husband is astounded that we both shed a pound or two, even as we seem to eat more. The trick: We walk *a lot.*

Walking is an essential part of the French way of life, and the average French woman walks three times as much as the average American. For the whole lower half of your body, there could be no better exercise: you work the legs top to bottom and the buttocks, particularly if your strides are long. And the cardiovascular benefits of brisk walking have been shown to be as good as those of running, but without endangering your joints.

I urge you to increase your walking in two ways:

First, add regular "dedicated" walks to your day. Not death marches, just smart strolls. Start small, if you like, then make your strolls a little longer each day. Whether it's walking to work all or part of the way, or for twenty minutes after dinner (good for digestion and unwinding), adding three hours of walking to your week is a painless and reliable way to weight loss. When you begin to see it working for you, you'll find yourself automatically walking more. Wherever I am, I begin most days with a twenty-minute walk before breakfast.

Second, look for ways to increase your "incidental" walk time. This means resisting the American impulse to save a step. We French are not as fiendish about finding shortcuts as Americans are. Perhaps it is why we are no longer a great power, but the trade-off is that we are not fat. In life, we believe the journey is the destination. If you're not that philosophical, remember it simply: Time saved equals calories not burned. Have a little walk around while waiting for someone (as we say, *faire les cent pas*, literally, "walk a hundred steps").

Contrary to popular wisdom, walking is not as simple as chewing gum. Any physical activity must be pursued thoughtfully, with an eye to balance and harmony. So, what is the best way to walk? Avoid treading congested streets and carrying heavy things. (Even if you can manage that bag, its weight creates a subconscious incentive to avoid walking next time.) Stilettos are not a good idea, but you don't need garish running shoes, either. French women wear comfortable loafers, pumps, or rubber-soled lace-ups that are presentable anywhere. City parks and roads without traffic in the country are great places to walk, but even the air-conditioned mall will do fine if being outdoors is not bearable where you are. I know an eighty-eight-year-old woman who lives in the suburbs, and all winter long she takes a daily walk in a huge supermarket. To each her own. Of course, city or country, you'll probably come to know your walk preferences only if you pay attention. Some respond to nature, others to people-watching. Discover what engages you.

The most important aspects of walking are posture and breathing. It's vital to hold your head erect and keep your back straight, chin up, as though your attention is fixed on some point in the distance or on looking for a lover in a foggy train station. But watch your step, too. (I know people who've found a lot of change in the street just looking down from time to time.) Relax your shoulders, then arch them back (feels like pushing out your chest), such that you can imagine a little brook running down your back between your shoulder blades, and be conscious of keeping them in that position. After a while, it becomes automatic. Bad posture in walking will announce itself with a sore neck and back.

Inhale and exhale deeply and slowly; concentrating on your breathing will improve the meditative value of your walk. As with eating, awareness heightens the overall stimulation of the experience, and stimulation equals satisfaction. Your gait is important, too: use your arms, and don't walk on the ball of the foot only; heel and toe is the way to go. *Always* carry and drink water. Before you know it, you'll be there.

On weekdays during my first two student years in Paris, I used to walk between the Eiffel Tower and the Sorbonne, a different route going and coming (though avoiding pastry shops each way while that was still necessary). On the weekends, my roommate and I, both provincial girls discovering Paris with very wide eyes, would spend Saturdays walking the different arrondissements or gardens or along the banks of the Seine. Often we must have walked six to eight miles, stopping only for lunch and a five o'clock ice cream—that little weekly reward—at the famous Berthillon on the Île St. Louis. In the end, we knew the city better than most Parisians.

For me, walking remains the ultimate time for freedom of thought. It's when I feel my tensions liberated and a kind of *bien-être*, as the promenade of the mind follows that of the body. It can be a special kind of indulgence, these moments when one becomes aware of really existing, as the images, information, and other sensations the world tries to press upon us all recede. Learning to be comfortable in that space, when it's just you, takes practice. But doing so diminishes the impulse to lie to yourself or run away. You won't want to.

Let's not forget the third dimension of earthly movement.

It always astounds me to see people who live no higher than the fourth floor taking the elevator. In France, walking up and down stairs is part of everyone's day. Unless you have a lot to carry, you wouldn't think of taking the elevator for a couple of flights. And often you have no choice, as in Paris, which is full of old buildings without elevators.

Of course, no one climbs stairs for an hour over a normal day, but think about this: The body spends about 60 calories an hour sleeping; if you swim, you'll do better at 430 calories; but climbing stairs consumes a stunning 1,100 calories per hour. *Vive l'escalier!*

In my third year as a student in Paris, I had the good fortune to become an apartment sitter for a painter who spent most of her time in the lovely southern town of Collioure. She offered me a room of my own, as well as free run of the rest of her huge place. I had major party visions, especially on seeing that wraparound terrace looking onto the Sorbonne and the lovely Square Painlevé (whose name means "Leavened Bread"!) next to the precious Cluny Museum of Medieval Art. It was a fantasy location, where the Fifth Arrondissement (Latin Quarter) borders the Sixth (St. Germain-des-Prés). There was only one catch: It was a sixth-floor walk-up.

When I moved in I had already shed the pounds I'd gained as an exchange student, but if I hadn't, my house-sitting stint would have made a big dent in the problem before long: I found myself losing weight without even meaning to—particularly during the May–June exam period, when I would go up and down all day, downstairs to study in the tiny Square Painlevé, then back upstairs for lunch or to use the bathroom or get another book I needed or my notebook for class around the corner. I managed to go up and down the eighty-nine (counting them became a private game) stairs six or eight times a day. By the beginning of the summer, I was floating in my clothes (despite my daily dose of chocolate and bread and lots of restaurant meals with friends), and when I put on my bikini in July, the change in shape, courtesy of *le grand escalier,* was a thrill. Better leg and buttock toning a trainer could not have delivered. That's when I became hooked on stairs, and now I seek them out, as religiously as most American women I know avoid them.

When I moved to New York, we first lived on the fourth floor of a West Village brownstone. I'll never forget opening the door for our first dinner guests, each of them, regardless of age, totally breathless from the three flights. These days we live on the fifteenth floor of a fifteen-story building (with elevator, *bien sûr*), so no one needs to walk up for a visit. But as my perplexed neighbors can verify, several times a week I can be seen going up and down the stairs (125—I still count) *sans problème.* The blackout of August 2003 was a revealing occasion for me. I was passing exhausted twenty-five- and forty-year-olds who'd stopped to rest on the sixth or eighth or tenth floor. Our building, I hasten to add, has a gym for its residents. Another case of the props of fitness standing in for results.

It strikes me as an American paradox: a nation with so many great athletes and a fascination for sports and such a mania for exercise technology, and they somehow avoid the easy, unheroic path to fitness. Sometimes I believe all these machines are a vestige of Puritanism: instruments of public self-flagellation to make up for private sins of couch riding and overeating. French women happily don't suffer from those extremes of good and evil. Wellness is a gray area of balance.

Simple as it may seem to add a few steps, it may be impractical for you or, for some reason, against your doctor's advice. (Always ask a physician first when it comes to exercise.) In that case, there are other ways of increasing the calorie-burn *quotidien* that should also do the trick. As with eating, it's a matter of compensation, and a good place to look is in the realm of so-called modern conveniences. Many things designed to make life easier, from remote control to no-iron sheets, have really only made us more sedentary. Studies show that the Amish are much less likely to get fat than other Americans. If you stop seeing repetitive chores as drudge work and instead look at them as a meditative form of mild exertion, you will be helping the weight-loss and wellness cause in a big way. Again, pick something you find rewarding. Cleaning house, believe it or not, can enhance your mood. It represents a job done, a kind of simple satisfaction in a world in which our tasks are more and more complex and our projects drag on for weeks.

Don't be deceived by the American tendency to view mundane exercise as strictly for people too old or weak for extreme training. Women of all ages can benefit enormously from more routine exertion. Also remember that you can increase or decrease depending on the results you see. Being a French woman requires continual fine-tuning. Practice it and soon you won't need to give it a second thought.

EASY MOVEMENTS AND EXERCISES

I'm not wistful for the era of daylong backbreaking work on the French farm. But I do believe that we have gone too far in developing a less physical lifestyle. Often the time saved is spent brooding about work and family, stewing in our juices.

Careful routine exertion can see you perfectly well through middle age, but as a woman gets older, there is a natural weakening of muscle and bone, and you may consider a bit of more special strength-training. Colette, who worked out madly, seems to have burned out early, and in her old age she was not very fit, couldn't even walk on her own. Small free weights (three to five pounds) used in simple, familiar exercises are a good way to preserve upper body tone and bone density and supplement the cardiovascular benefits of an active lifestyle. It's also good as we age to attend to our abdomen with a few sit-ups first thing in the morning—it's never too early to start doing so, as they are the muscles that hold all the vital organs in place, in addition to their support of good posture.

You can incorporate simple resistance movements into your daily routine even before you leave the house. After your shower or bath, for instance, try to dry your toes with your towel while keeping your legs straight. While waiting in your car or in the subway, contract your abs for twelve seconds with your back pressed against the seat (better for you than road rage). Use your own body weight as resistance wherever possible: isometric exercises, discreet but effective, are very French. When reading a magazine at home, try sitting on the floor with your legs stretched and apart in a V and your hands on each side; this is a great stretch for your inner thigh muscles. At work, get up from your desk periodically (people are amazed to see a CEO doing her own photocopying, but it's an excuse for me to walk to the end of the hall and stretch). You get the picture. The key is to increase daily energy expenditure. Add a few moves to the regular ones all day long. Don't save your steps, multiply them. Little changes are always easier than big ones, but they do add up. Take the long view: burning a mere fifty extra calories a day through *les petites choses* (little things) equals a few pounds of fat a year. *Faites simple* and you'll never cry out, "I give up!"

À BOUT DE SOUFFLE (BREATHLESS)

In the end, all movements depend on proper breathing, the one movement we do more than any other (twenty-two thousand times a day). It takes some calories to move fifteen kilos of air each day, as we do. Breathlessness will stop you in your tracks and prevent the body's efficient burning of fuel. Moreover, steady breathing with awareness promotes a balanced appreciative relationship to food. You may consider yourself an accomplished breather, but it's worth your while to learn how to do it better.

That's what I told a group of women as I opened a three-day business seminar in San Francisco about ten years ago. I showed them a few techniques I learned from an instructor in Paris. I didn't care if they never tried them again. The point is that no one should go through life without being made to think at least once about the deep significance of breathing. And if you continue thinking about it, you can harness the most discreet and portable mechanism we have for reestablishing the mind-body link, which is so terribly eroded by our fast-paced lives.

Conscious breathing is the easiest form of meditation and the most basic part of yoga, which I highly recommend if you have the inclination to take classes in anything. This type of breathing disconnects eating from our stress-response equipment, a major cause of overeating and bingeing. It also enhances our overall energy by releasing energy in every cell of the body. Breathing is the driving process of metabolism.

I practice breathing movements in the subway (okay, not too deeply there), on the plane, lying in bed, and sitting at my desk, but also as part of my home routine—wherever I have to breathe, anyway. Part of the appeal is being in the moment. Breathing is the ultimate present-moment stimulation. Think about doing it, and you don't think of the past or the future. You are in the "here and now." That's the ultimate zone diet.

Try these basics.

Step 1: Rhythm and Awareness

Close your eyes. Place one hand on your belly and notice your breathing. Feel your hand rise slightly with each new breath in. Feel it fall with each breath out. Focus on this motion of rising and falling for 12 breaths.

Step 2: Countdown to Sleep

Start with the Step 1 movement until you are comfortable with the pace. As you breathe in, inwardly say "twelve," then breathe out. With the next breath say "eleven," breathe out. Continue until you reach zero. Take your time; slow is good. Repeat this for a couple of minutes . . . or until you fall asleep.

Step 3: Slowdown to Sleep

Now when you breathe in count to 6 to yourself, and when you breathe out count to 9. While you do it, clear your mind of any thoughts and concentrate totally on your breathing. It takes only a few repetitions or deep breaths until you feel relaxed, and eventually you will fall asleep.

Step 4: Wave Breathing

Digestion depends on the autonomic system, which explains the influence our emotions have on our gastric function. Therefore it is essential to breathe well in order to eat more slowly and to give the brain the necessary time to register satiety. The wave is best practiced when you are, or think you are, hungry and/or before meals.

Standing, sitting, or lying flat on your back, put one hand on your belly and the other above it midchest, wrist below the breasts. Breathe in and expand your chest while pushing a bit on the abdomen. Breathe out and expand your abdomen while exerting a slight pressure on the chest. Repeat 24 times, then go back to your normal breathing before you return to whatever you were doing.

Step 5: Alternate Nostril Breathing

A little odd, but bear with me—French is a very nasal language. Standing or sitting, breathe out through both nostrils. Next close your right nostril with your right thumb. Breathe in on the left side. Close your left nostril with the right index finger. (Both nostrils are now pinched closed.) Hold breath in. Release thumb and exhale out of right nostril, breathe in again through right nostril. Hold and again close nostril with right thumb. Release index finger and breathe out left side. This completes 1 set. Repeat 6 times. Count to 6 for each holding, breathing in, breathing out.

Step 6: Yawning

I actually learned this one when I first moved to New York and was studying modern dance as a hobby. I was no great dancer, but I was a star at yawning and can do it on cue without any difficulty. Before that class, I never knew it relieves stress, calms you down, and even puts you to sleep, if repeated, which sometimes happened at the end of the class as we lay on our backs, practicing the art of yawning. While you yawn, you actually allow a greater amount of oxygen than normal into your lungs, which revitalizes blood flow. Even the sound of a good yawn helps reduce tension. To make yourself yawn, you have to breathe in deeply and stretch your mouth open as wide as possible. After two or three tries, the natural yawning response is triggered and can go on indefinitely.

DORMEZ-VOUS?

The question is not just for *frère* Jacques. Sleep is the most neglected state of being in American life. We think we can cut corners, push ourselves to the limit. To some degree, it has even become subject to the calculus of good and evil, with virtue ascribed to making do with less. This is nonsense. Nothing else except breathing and drinking water is as immediately vital to our well-being as sleep. And there is an underacknowledged connection between sleeping too little and gaining weight.

Proust began his masterpiece with a slow and agonized wind-down to z's. He gave it a lot of thought and comment, as we French will do with most things. Now, while we don't wish to encourage such performance anxiety, sleep must be done well. There is an art to this, too. But as with other pleasures—and good sleep is one of the most basic—respect for the individual is paramount, as no two of us have the same requirements or patterns.

When we lived and labored according to the sun and the seasons, getting to sleep was easier, and our internal clock (circadian rhythms) reset itself reliably as the days got longer or shorter. Now each of us follows her own clock, often getting by with too little sleep. At the same time, there is an insomnia epidemic, with a corresponding wave of pharmaceutical remedies. We are regularly warned of the mounting national "sleep debt" that research has demonstrated increases insulin resistance and triggers the release of stress-response hormones. It's a vicious cycle, since the body's responses to sleep deprivation can make it only harder for us to sleep. Sleeplessness also makes us listless, which encourages us to overeat, food being the most obvious other way to achieve reinvigoration. When we feel this way, we tend to lean on high-energy foods. And of course, lack of sleep interferes with the mental mechanisms by which we register pleasure. Optimal experience depends on sensory alertness. Consider a good night's sleep vital to proper eating and balance.

There are rituals that can promote a good night's rest. To me, the tisane is essential. But water in any form can help, because dehydration always undermines the quality of our sleep time. For this reason, alcohol just before sleep is not good and in small amounts is known to have the "paradoxical effect" of being a stimulant. (We French only *seem* to have a monopoly on paradox.)

As to setting, look around your bedroom: you don't need to be a feng shui master to make improvements. Gentle lighting that promotes somnolence can help greatly. In Provence in summer, the bloom of lavender delivers a natural sleep aid into the night air. I'm always reminded of the splendid lavender fields of the Abbaye de Sénanque, near Gordes in the Vaucluse. The smell is wonderfully soporific, and you can enjoy it in the freshly picked variety or by burning a bit of the plant's essential oil. Louis XIV demanded the presence of all his worthies in his bedchamber not only for his *coucher* (going-to-bed ritual), but also for his *lever* (rising). You don't need an audience to practice routines that tell your body bedtime approaches.

Try to go to bed relaxed. We French like eating late but don't go to bed without having digested dinner. This may mean eating lightly at night (when carbohydrates are a good idea) with a glass of wine (a relaxant if used in moderation and with food). Better to have a yogurt snack just before bed to neutralize the occasional *coup de faim* than to eat too late or overeat early and fall asleep on a full stomach. Controlled breathing is another way to prepare your body. The yawning exercise is useful here. Don't neglect room temperature, either; even in winter this should be cool, sixty-eight degrees at maximum. Except in blizzard conditions, do open your window a crack for some fresh air.

It's important to catch the train when it's in the station. If you ignore sleepiness signals, you may need another two hours to feel sleepy again. Sleeping and rising at the same time each day is a good idea. The ritual of sleeping until noon on Sundays "to catch up" is based on a misconception. Food may be organized on the weekly calendar, but not sleep. Better to try napping ten to twenty minutes during the day (avoid the long siesta of two hours, as it will interfere with your sleep rhythm). Finally, remember moderation. While need can vary from one individual to another, less than six hours or more than eight may be unhealthy. Though few of us sleep too much, it is possible to have too much of even this good thing. Your body will sleep less efficiently if you give it too much time *au lit.*

POSTURE

A little plug for good posture. Weight is related to height, or at least our sense of it. French women learn to hold their chin high and have good posture (just pretend you have a rope or wire attached to the center of your head, pulling you up). For some reason, only girls get the *tiens-toi droite* (stand up straight) reminder as we grow up. I recall one at the *lycée* who stood so erect that we asked her what she had been doing. At home her mother would hold a ruler across her shoulders to force her to memorize the right posture. When I was growing up, we learned to practice posture in ballet class. None of us became ballerinas, but the few classes did help. And our gym teacher always advised that as we French were a smallish race, cheating to look *quelques centimètres plus grandes* was no crime. So when I catch myself slouching while sitting in front of the computer or walking on the street, I think about the gym teacher and correct my posture instantly. And I do feel taller.

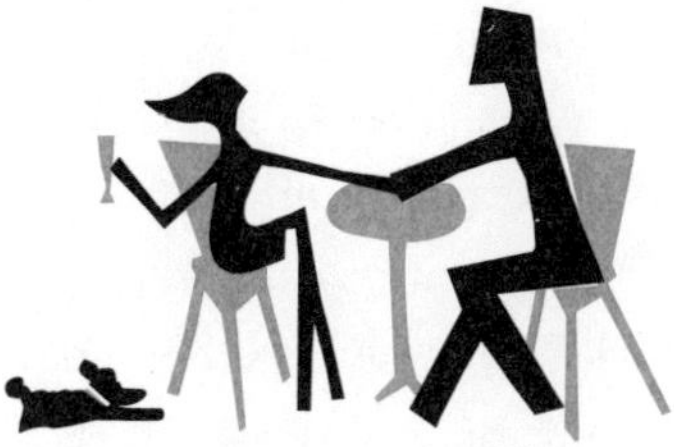

11

STATES OF DESIRE

The mind is the French woman's ultimate firewall against getting fat, and the senses are, of course, the portals to the mind. Through them we take in the world—its flavors, its textures, its sounds, and its smells. We all practice a little form of "yoga" with our senses. We concentrate on them just as we concentrate on our breathing. In this way we get the most out of experience, including what we eat. Contentment of this kind is something you make for yourself. It's the essence of *l'art de vivre* (the art of living), which is how we French pursue *joie de vivre* (the joy of living). While this pursuit sometimes causes us to be mocked as "too bourgeois," in fact, our way of pursuing pleasure has little to do with social status. Our next vacation means much more to us than a new car, and we would never sacrifice the former for the latter except in a case of dire necessity. Give us *being* and *feeling* over *having* any day.

Anyone possessed of the five human senses can reap the benefits of sharpening them. Walking on the beach, touching a pet, eating an orange, picking up and sniffing a piece of wood—all are sensory experiences of which we can become more aware through practice. Concentrate on each, develop your own terms of description, and soon your every moment will be fuller. One must never forget that little experiences produce, through association and memory, a gamut of emotions. These are linked with our life experiences, culture, and environment. Proust's madeleine takes countless forms. The more conscious you become of these effects, the more you can make of them. And the better you'll be at evading the effects of more destructive emotions.

French women make sure they have lots of *petits riens*, those little nothings of daily pleasure that are actually quite something to us. We have so many words for pampering— *gâter, dorloter, bichonner, se chouchouter*—but we don't equate it with decadence. It makes us enjoy life more, from moment to moment, and keeps us from seeking too much consolation from any one pleasure, such as food. If we deny ourselves something, it's not to teach our greedy selves a lesson. (Self-punishment is never our path to well-being.) The only purpose of withholding some pleasure is so we can more fully enjoy everything else for having it in proper balance.

Of course, there's nothing we enjoy as often or universally as food. So it's quite foreign to us the way Americans associate eating with sin and guilt. A French woman might refer to her afternoon pastry at a café terrace as her *petit péché mignon,* but she is being ironic (only in the French mind could sin be "tiny" and "adorable"!). The American gastronomic morality, by contrast, is dead serious. As the charming Anglo-sometime-American Francophile Peter Mayle writes in *French Lessons,* "Scarcely a week goes by without some ominous pronouncement about the price we must pay for our brief moments of indulgence." The trouble, as he wisely understands, is not having a little butter and wine and red meat; the trouble is having way too much. Eating in America has become controversial behavior, with all sorts of "non-nutritional" sexual, social, political, cultural, and even clinical overtones. Our troubles with weight have as much to do with our attitudes toward eating as they do with what we are ingesting. We are seeing a growing psychosis that I believe actually adds stress to our already stressful way of life. It is fast erasing the simple values of pleasure. Without a national change of heart, we have little hope of turning the tide of the obesity epidemic.

THE LOVE OF EATING

For the French, Colette put it best when she described the table as *un rendez-vous d'amour et d'amitié* (a date with love and friendship). And it's not a purely figurative description, because we tend to see our pleasures as being interconnected. We can't imagine anything more boring than to live with someone who doesn't care about food or eating or sharing meals. One passion goes hand in hand with another. Of course, it's a two-way street. The actor Omar Sharif captivated a generation of French females not only with his dark good looks in *Dr. Zhivago,* but also by declaring he could not desire a woman who didn't love to eat. Certainly French women, suckers though we may be for the intellectual type, could hardly care for a man indifferent to sensuality.

Sensuality is vital to our ideas of seduction, and seduction figures prominently in the French woman's sense of herself. We have always known one doesn't have to be a great beauty to seduce, but one does have to be sensual. A model may catch a man's eye, but if she happens to be a sensually abstinent woman, she won't hold him for long. Style, a sense of taste, and elegance can go far, too, but pure arm candy is an unsatisfying supper. It's not that French women are not assaulted with as many unnatural ideals of womanhood presented in glossy magazines; we just don't take it personally. No matter how well turned out or fit, if one is not *bien dans sa peau,* one can never project that certain *état de grâce.* This is something every woman can learn to achieve, and French women channel more intuitively than most. For all her attention to what she wears and what she eats, a French woman is most defined by ease in being herself and the attractiveness of taking her pleasures. It has little to do with weighing a certain amount. And it doesn't come upon you through avoiding food.

Au contraire, the meal itself, in all its splendor, has been a scene of seduction since the grand court dinners of Versailles. French women seduce with the way they order and savor food, with the sly complicity of stealing a taste from the other's plate or feeding our lover a particularly choice morsel. And just as certain formalities at the table can heighten the psychic zing of the food, so too can setting, presentation, and ambiance intensify the mood of dining together. A surprise dish or unplanned dinner out can pique the curiosity more than the loveliest routine supper. I always recommend throwing in a bottle of Champagne as the clincher. For the French, the sex appeal of eating is second nature. Perhaps this is why so many erotic blandishments refer to food. I grew up hearing the entire repertoire of edible endearments: *mon petit canard* (my little duck), *mon chou* (cabbage), *ma tourterelle* (dove), *ma caille* (quail) . . .

UNE AMOUREUSE RIGOLOTE

Sex itself is a great antiaging formula with no side effects. It has cardiovascular benefits and increases the production of hormones that diminish stress and improve mood. A good mood is the right state in which to enjoy all pleasures properly, especially food. The right frame of mind is vital to contentment, diminishing the urge for excess. But even more than sex, being in love is good for you. Gauguin in Tahiti created a wood relief he entitled *Soyez Amoureuse pour Être Heureuse* (To Be Happy Be in Love). Not a bad recipe.

Perhaps this sounds to you like one of those "easier said than done" prescriptions, on a par with "Eat right and exercise." Nevertheless, I observe many women failing to embrace love as pleasure. Relationships and marriage can be pursued with the same grim determination that some bring to their careers. (There has even been a recent book about applying MBA training to finding a husband.) Romance is not a science but an art, no less so than the art of eating well. And it takes cultivation and refinement if a relationship is to offer its fullest rewards.

In love we blend versatility with constancy, the stiff and

the supple, the excitement of glamour with the pleasure of comfort—contrasts and surprises that keep love as well as food interesting. And we are not careless with our investments, as usual favoring quality over quantity. True love depends on truly knowing someone, and getting to know someone takes a very long while, often a lifetime. Perhaps this is why French women are better than any others I know at preserving spark and mystery even after ten, twenty, or more years of cohabitation! It's worth the money and effort. I am always reminded of Louis Aragon, who said, in what is probably my favorite love poem, *"Il n'y a pas d'amour heureux / Mais c'est notre amour à tous deux,"* which translates loosely as "There is no happy love / But the love of us two."

Nothing promotes the continued spontaneity of love like laughter. French women dream of finding *un amoureux rigolo* (a love who is funny, makes us laugh). The old wisdom that laughter keeps us young finds empirical support in the fact that a four-year-old laughs about five hundred times a day, while for the average adult it's only fifteen. If that's your idea of growing up, you can keep it. The French woman understands intuitively that one does not laugh because one is happy; one is happy because one laughs. It's both a physical and psychic pleasure: it is relaxing, stimulating, liberating, and sensual. It's a pleasant response to emotion that heightens the emotion itself. The physical act of laughing stimulates the production of hormones that elevate mood; it's also a form of internal calisthenic that improves blood circulation and, yes, does burn more calories than sitting glumly. Laughs are like wild mushrooms: they don't deliver themselves to you—you have to go in search of them, whether by pursuing the unexpected or by being totally crazy (*dingue* is the word we use), to keep the adventure of living adventurous. Whether in friendship or in romance, one shouldn't sit around waiting to be entertained. Take the initiative and make a rendezvous with someone whose company you enjoy. Don't let a busy life or electronic communication gadgets be your excuse for excess solitude—it's a talent, but a rare one, to be able to make yourself laugh.

Years ago Edward's mother, who lucky for me adores me, was much relieved when he finally proposed. But she knew for certain we'd remain together when later she'd ask him how it was going and Edward would say, "She makes me laugh." In fact, at holiday meals, I enjoy making his entire family laugh. Over the years we've laughed a lot, and when I ask him, "Do you still love me?" he always answers, "As long as you make me laugh." I make sure I do.

Dr. Miracle was first to tell me: "*Tout est une question d'attitude*" ("Everything's a matter of attitude"). The great Provençal writer Marcel Pagnol believed that God gave laughter to human beings as consolation for being intelligent. I prefer to believe he made us intelligent so we could appreciate a good laugh.

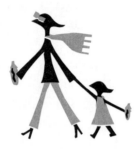

12

LIFE STAGES

Reaching and maintaining equilibrium is not done by force of heredity; it's something we cultivate through the way we live. Genetics plays a part, of course, and balance certainly does seem easier for some. But looks can be deceiving; some may actually mask unhealthy habits. Consider the proverbial model who eats nothing but burgers and pizza yet doesn't gain an ounce. Genetics may be protecting her insides—for now— from this assault (if not from our envious glares). But just as likely, such a woman may in fact be less well than one who must pay much more attention to what she consumes, how much she moves, and so forth. Genetic predisposition to slenderness is not, as I have said, disproportionately distributed among French women. Most who appear to live in healthy balance are actually working at it. But that work has been made infinitely easier by wise cultural conditioning and practice.

Unfortunately for all women—see under "Life, unfairness of"—the equilibrium we work to achieve shifts as we age. If we don't continue paying close attention to our bodies, our healthy balance will be pulled out from under us. But despair not: attention and incremental adjustment throughout life are easier than big corrections following long intervals of imbalance. Alertness and rapid response can allow us to enjoy a long life of pleasures while never getting fat.

Still, it does happen. We can be eating well and staying active for years when, bang!—force majeure. This is true for all humans, but especially for women, whose weight and silhouette can be radically altered by three major physiological and psychological events, in which hormones run amuck: adolescence, pregnancy, and menopause. All three present a serious potential for troublesome weight gain, and it's better to plan for them than to eat first and ask questions later.

But let's begin at the beginning.

BIRTH TO AGE SEVEN

While this could hardly be mistaken for a child-care book, common sense tells us that habits acquired young are the hardest to break. Take advantage of the last moment when you have complete control over what your child consumes. As children we develop our lifelong sense of what is natural and comforting, and the adult continues to seek comfort from the same sources, regardless of how unhealthful. You needn't read the complete Proust to figure this out. The best gift you can give a child is a conditioned attraction to the things that are good for her. First and foremost, this means water.

Beware of dehydration among infants. The critical period is the first two years, especially the first six months. A baby's body is 65 to 80 percent water (versus 60 percent for an adult). Without plenty of water, a baby, especially one kept too warm, can dehydrate in as little as three hours, a problem only exacerbated by the common infant problems of vomiting and diarrhea. When a baby refuses to drink, sleeps too much, is sluggish, has a gray complexion, or breathes too fast, it's time to get oral rehydration salts at the pharmacy. Don't let things get that far. Make sure your infant is well hydrated. Baby food is usually rich in water, but the taste for water by itself won't develop naturally if you limit a baby's liquids to juice and milk. (Perhaps the questionable preference for caloric liquids over water starts here.)

Eating well is something that needs to be taught early, but as everyone knows, a baby's palate is no more well developed than its teeth. Don't try to start too early with intense flavors and turn your baby off. By the time a child is three years old, however, French mothers start cultivating good taste.

Especially in the Western world, children have many noxious eating temptations, foods chemically treated to trick our evolutionary programming into believing they are good eats. You may need to fight fire with fire, fooling kids, as I was fooled, into eating what is good until they can appreciate for themselves. Americans seem less inclined to do this than they were fifty years ago; they seem to believe any form of deceit in child rearing will lead to trauma. This is nonsense. There's nothing wrong with fooling kids into learning which foods are good and which are not to be abused. Take time to develop some games that make this easier. When I was a girl, my father would come home for lunch (as most workers and school-children did in those days) and we would play *pèle la pomme*—peel the apple. My mother didn't like the skins, so my father was assigned the peeling, which we watched him do with wonderful dexterity as we spoke about the morning's goings-on.

Nutrition should be taught at school, but too often it is not, and by then it can be harder to change habits ingrained by supermarkets and fast-food chains and virtually everything on television—mostly they are selling not healthy eating, but products supposed to be edible, a term I use advisedly. Few are selling naturally good food. I was amazed as an exchange student in Weston, Massachusetts, to discover frozen dinners. Now many of them even carry claims of being "healthy options." A meal that can be packed and frozen and thawed is nothing you should desire—much less teach your kids to want.

In France, where globalization has only started to precipitate a previously unimaginable obesity wave among small kids, a nationwide school program of nutritional awareness has been implemented (big government has its uses). It also helps that there is not nearly as much variety on television and TV plays a much smaller role in the average French child's life, sparing her the roughly ten thousand food ads the average American child sees annually. Food on television makes one think about eating and gets one's gastric juices flowing, triggering the release of insulin, lowering one's blood sugar, and stimulating food cravings. It's gastronomic pornography.

Here are some basic rules your kids will thank you for when they become adults who aren't fat:

- Get your children used to drinking water straight (not juice or "fruitlike" drinks or soda) as their thirst quencher. As in adults, thirst is a faulty indicator of proper hydration, kicking in only when the tank is way too low. Kids should learn to pay attention to their urine. If it's not pale and clear, more water is needed.

- Now is the time to learn the meaning of three meals a day and sensible portions—a hungry child's eyes can be bigger than her stomach, as we say. Some kids just can't bear food in the morning, but the French agree with most experts that classroom attention and learning are markedly improved by a real breakfast. Making sure your kids eat at regular intervals will reduce the menace of snacking, which usually means junk to kids left to their own devices.

- Teach your children the rituals of civilized eating by setting a good example. Don't eat in front of the TV if you don't want them to. Dinner is a ritual; table conversation is an art—even if it amounts to playing *mange ta soupe* as our *nounou,* Yvette, did.

- Expose them to the widest variety of vegetables and fruits, showing them how good things can be in season. Tasteless fruits and vegetables won't win them over for life.

- Learn to use treats. There is nothing wrong with the old custom of rewarding good eating, whether in adults or in children. But never use junk as a reward. And try to instill low-sugar tolerance. A dessert doesn't have to be super-sweet to be a treat. Try a *tarte aux fruits.* Most kids' cereals have more sugar than a French pastry; avoid them like the plague. (I wonder how many children on behavior-modifying pharmaceuticals are merely sugar junkies.)

- Don't stock bad foods out of convenience. But always have something to snack on. Kids love tangerines, grapes. Did you know raw fennel makes a great snack food?
- Get them involved in food preparation—looking, smelling, and tasting ingredients: what you're doing in the kitchen shouldn't be a mystery to them. Take them to food markets, gardens, and farms where they can pick fruit.
- Don't be a permissive parent. Fear that their kids won't like them has terrorized lots of Americans. The French are more traditional in child rearing and accept that children benefit from structure and strictures.
- Get your kids moving. Apart from those committed to sports lessons and teams, exertion for many American kids has been reduced to the virtual kind of the Playstation, fine for hand-eye coordination but no substitute for the real thing. Kids have much more energy than adults; without proper outlets, emotional problems, including overeating, can result. In Europe, you see kids playing outside till dinner—as they used to in America in the days before the obesity epidemic.
- Remember: children imitate their parents, so practice good manners and habits for wellness. Also remember that prevention in all things starts in childhood.

AGES SEVEN TO SEVENTEEN

Above all, getting enough calcium is critical during this period, when 40 to 50 percent of the definitive bone capital is constituted. Be on the alert—many girls avoid dairy products because they view them as fattening. This is a big mistake.

Yogurt and cheese should be eaten regularly. Now is also the time when girls learn their taste for coffee and sodas, sugar and caffeine, so encourage moderation.

A few more "rules" and suggestions for the formative years, when weight may become an issue for the first time in our lives:

- Some teenage girls are drawn to vegetarianism nowadays, which has both advantages and liabilities. It's not to be discouraged, as long as proteins, especially dairy, are consumed. But if your kids are carnivores, like most French children, it's a good time to establish the principle that one should have meat only two to three times a week. Teach them the pleasures of seafood in various forms. Nowadays some kids love sushi, which wasn't an option when I was growing up.
- Start teaching them how to cook simple dishes, the sooner the better. Connection to preparing one's food is the French woman's lifeline to healthy eating. So is cleaning up.
- Movement. Don't trust school athletic programs as the only source of exertion. Half the gym class can be wasted suiting up and taking attendance. If your kid is an athlete, that's great; but if not, sitting around until dinner is not an option. Chores, volunteer work, and many other activities build character and burn calories. Don't run a hotel for your kids; make sure they pick up after themselves.
- Now is the time to grow up respecting our liquid assets. Eight to ten glasses of water a day may be an easier sell when you explain the benefits in weight control and keep-

ing the complexion clear. They'll need even more if they sneak salty snack foods. I also recommend that parents be the first to serve alcohol (preferably in the form of wine and water) to kids and teach them respectful use. This is not something they should be prowling around to obtain behind your back.

In general, bodies still developing need to eat a bit of everything. For perfect nutrition, children and teenagers should really be having about twenty different foods a day. Well, we must do what we can. If there is difficulty with meat or fish, there are plenty of ways to "fool" the wary youngster, from rolling prunes in veal or turkey scaloppine to hiding veggies in an omelet and serving fish dipped in an egg batter and cooked in a nonstick pan. Barter once in a while. On Wednesdays, my parents often served *biftek de cheval* (horse steak), which I loathed mostly for sentimental reasons, though the meat is actually quite tasty. It was always followed with a small surprise dessert. So I ate my horse.

The increase in body fat that accompanies adolescence generally falls in the middle of the seven-to-seventeen period. It's time for every young woman, French or otherwise, to get some counsel from a family doctor or even a gynecologist. Professionals can confirm with more credibility that a bit of weight gain is natural and healthy. Proper menstrual function depends on fat reserves. In thin girls, puberty is often delayed; in not-so-thin girls, it can be precocious. But if weight problems do occur, the most important countermeasure is the three-meals-a-day system. There is no surer ballast for physical and mental well-being at this time. Girls who have had the golden rules of proper nutrition programmed into them will be better able to fend for themselves when they leave the nest.

AGES SEVENTEEN TO THIRTY-FIVE

For many, the twenties seem like the time of infinite possibility, although in retrospect a woman will always idealize her thirties. Late teens and early twenties are inevitably a tough transition, as they were for me: college, starting a career, even a family. This great stress comes just as we have already exhausted everyone's patience with teenage angst. I've met countless women in their twenties suffering weight problems because of not yet having grown into adult habits of eating, drinking, and moving. It's particularly painful to see them suckered by unsustainable diets—to which faith in technology, common in today's youth, appears to make them especially vulnerable. A little fuzzy science is a dangerous thing. They also tend to want results timed to social events, of which there are many for the predominantly single demographic. So the idea of ten pounds in two weeks is extremely seductive. Making matters worse, most haven't learned anything about cooking. If this is you, I recommend the French woman's Full Monty: a month of nutritional inventory, Magical Leek Soup, short- and long-term recasting. Now is the time to get serious about putting away childish things.

The freedom most enjoy during the seventeen-to-thirty-five period can also invite seemingly grown-up excesses: rich meals out (for business and adult courtship rituals) and especially excess alcohol consumption among the freshly legal and unsupervised. For this demographic, most overeating occurs after eight p.m., when you should be most *en garde*. It's important to develop hunger pacifiers for the times leading up to lunch and dinner and the twilight zone before bed.

Muscle mass and bone density should be at their peak. Ironically, though, now is the time when most of us fall into a destructive sedentary lifestyle, fostered by the fact that more and more jobs require us to sit at a desk all day for the first time in our lives. The habits of movement, the principle of *faire les cent pas*, can be a help here, though the girl in us still wants to blast away her sins in StairMaster marathons. Eventually this gets too boring or exhausting, and the roof caves in on her precarious equilibrium. The sooner you learn the French woman's incremental approach, the easier and more pleasurable will be the rest of your life. Try to transform exercise time into entertainment; look for activities and exertions that amuse you, especially if you can do them with friends. There are a thousand stops on the road from triathlete to couch potato. It is an absolute must to start walking at least thirty minutes a day during these years. Swimming and yoga are also wonderful if you have the inclination. But in any case, you must not let attention to muscle tone and flexibility go until the next stage, when they will be much harder to recover. Ditto metabolism, which naturally declines beginning as early as twenty-five!

For pregnant women, fat accumulation is natural and tends to occur mainly in the first months to build the body's reserves for breast-feeding. The risk of postpartum weight problems is much greater if you are slightly overweight before you become pregnant. So before you start managing an equilibrium for two, it's a good idea to get your own in order.

Don't fall back on inevitability theory: "What's the use? In three months I'll be big as a house anyway."

Breast-feeding is good for the baby, but it's also good for the mother, putting the fat reserves to their intended use for milk production. A month of breast-feeding can do wonders trimming the silhouette, especially below the waist, reducing what we call *culottes de cheval* ("riding breeches," or saddle-bags); losing those pregnancy thighs is a true obsession with French women. The exertions of motherhood can be a great help if you manage the stress sensibly.

Here are some rules to live by as soon as you are running your own show, with or without others:

- Don't watch yourself become a Botero sculpture: react. A little initiative and discipline go a long way. Now that you are making choices as an adult for the first time, make sure they are adult choices. The rules you violate are no longer your mother's, and it's no longer simply a matter of not getting caught.
- Career progress, marriage, and motherhood can be particular stress factors in these years. Mistakes, doubts, and failures are bound to befall you. The best defense is learning to savor *les petits bonheurs*, all the little things that make each day a miracle, be it a sunrise on your way to work, a flowering bush in bloom, or an unexpected smile from a stranger. In facing challenges, aim to be the master, not the subject, of your life: choice and risk are intertwined; all roads to success run through such an awareness. Keep dreaming intensely (too many of us stop at this stage), but seize the day as well. How you learn to live now will set the stage for the rest of your life.

- Sources of fatigue and tension will multiply; combat them with physical activities, not cocktails. Discover new forms of movement—yoga, dance, golf, tennis, or anything that appeals to you—but don't neglect walking and stair-climbing.
- Tanning booth: NO! Sunglasses and sunscreen: YES! Think ahead: Better pale today than Botoxed tomorrow.
- Your metabolism is as high as it will ever be; enjoy it and don't be afraid to try new foods, but don't neglect fresh fruits and vegetables in season.
- Start paying attention to ingredients and what you are putting into your body. Even if you don't plan to be a chef, a cooking class can be fun and change your relationship to food for the better.

AGES THIRTY-FIVE TO FIFTY-FIVE

"Not older but wiser" is a hollow consolation only for those who expect it to be. French women are proverbially and in fact at their peak in these years—we truly believe it. You can, too. If you have cultivated well-being up to this point, you are primed to reap to full advantage the experience and awareness of your pleasures, including food and sex. At the same time, as you must know, there are agents provocateurs conspiring against your hard-won equilibrium, including greater responsibilities of work and family. This may be the time for caring for both parents and children—a big squeeze. Gone is much of our "free time." Even worse, we face a relatively rapid decline in metabolism. French women recognize this time as both peak and crunch, and the great majority do not surrender.

Denied youth's seemingly infinite forgiveness, you now

face the moment when lack of real commitment to healthy eating and living will show. It is no time for what mass-marketed diet programs offer. Even if you lose weight, you'll gain wrinkles and look gaunter as tissue loosens with rapid water loss. And sleep beckons as never before. Remember when you could stay out all night and still go to work looking okay? Adieu to all that. Sleep deprivation shows big-time in this stage and becomes a major contributor to weight gain. Just accept that the days of burning the candle at both ends with impunity are over. Beginning at thirty-five, think in terms of a "rule of seven." With every seven years hereafter, your body is changing enough to require an inventory and overhaul of habits. Don't wait for round-number birthdays, which can often induce paralysis and trauma just when everyone is watching. At thirty-five metabolism begins its slowdown, and you can't eat as you did in your twenties; if typical, you will start trading a half pound of muscle for a half pound of fat every year. At forty-two, hormone levels begin to drop until menopause at, say, forty-nine, when the serious loss of bone density also begins. For this reason, now is the time French women, lifelong walkers, also pick up weights. Resistance training is the surest way to reverse the muscle-to-fat trade-off that more than anything sets the twenty-somethings apart from their elders. It also retards bone loss and the slowdown in metabolism (remember, muscle burns more calories than other tissue types, even at rest). Now, you don't want to overdo it, as Colette unfortunately did. Start out with three- to five-pound weights, and favor slow movements controlled by your muscles through the full range of motion. Momentum does not tone your body; tone comes from slowly controlled reps. Muscle bulk comes only from more serious weights. If you discover the gym as something you can enjoy—never a necessity if you stick to small weights (safe at any speed) and keep up your walking and multiplying your little exertions—engage a trainer for at least a session or two. As I still detest gyms, I have no advice on the ever more complicated devices they offer—they look like weapons systems. While you treat the upper body with free weights, do morning sit-ups for the midsection. Do them religiously. And for the legs, I have but one word: stairs.

One mustn't underestimate the profound psychological and emotional impact of these years, especially if they include the very common traumas of divorce or losing a parent. It's a stage when thoughts inevitably turn to our own mortality, too. Either you can become morose, or you can apply your heightened awareness to cultivating pleasures. (I don't have to tell you which French women choose.) Having outgrown the youthful demand for immediate gratification puts you at an advantage for losing weight like a French woman. Also, having tried many things by this age, you know better than ever what delights and what doesn't. No one can appreciate little things as much as someone who has done a little living. But you can't ignore the debit column: the demands, even the reversals of fortune, may push you toward the zero degree of pleasures. Don't go there. If you can't name your pleasures, chances are you've surrendered too many of them. It's time to start cultivating.

For me, these years saw the introduction of new types of food. I now love soy nuts, whole soybeans roasted to a crunchy texture and nutty flavor. There has also been a slight decrease in portions and frequency of certain known "offend-ers." I've reduced my chocolate fix from daily to perhaps three times a week, and I also eat red meat less often. But doing it gradually, one doesn't notice a pinch. It's been during these years, too, that I have added the fifteen flights of stairs a few times a week to my scheduled walk. For me those twenty min-utes a day have been key to holding my ground.

Dr. Miracle advised that if you look healthy at twenty, that's more or less the weight you should keep for the rest of your life. Here are the basics for making that perfectly reason-able goal a reality:

- Increase your proportion of fruits and vegetables as com-pared with other food types, especially fatty and sugary ones, which you should aim to reduce anyway if you consume them frequently. Even a sweet tooth will re-equilibrate if conditioned slowly. Practice "less is more" more aggressively, avoiding meaningless calories and sav-ing them for real pleasures. Enjoy them with attention.
- Try to pay more attention to the rhythms of your life, daily, weekly, monthly. Bring a mental dimension to your physical movement. Awareness reduces stress and pro-motes a feeling of well-being. Practice more controlled breathing.
- Carry water everywhere you go, and increase your intake to at least two quarts a day.
- Start taking a multivitamin with food.
- Learn to say no, with an eye to saying yes to something else.
- Build small rest periods into your day. (I used to go to parties and dinners straight from work; now I go home

beforehand, take a shower, and do a few minutes of meditation. Result: I face the evening with renewed energy.) Take a breather at your desk: eyes closed and controlled breathing.

- Try to find new interests. Life seems fuller with novelties, and too many women depend on interests of their youth to see them through their middle years. Yesteryear's novelties may be today's rut. Relatively few of your possible activities have been closed to you on account of age. Curiosity, no less than openness to pleasure, is not the exclusive property of the young.

- Your skin will get dryer and lose some of its elasticity, but you don't need surgery or stem cell therapy. You do need plenty of moisturizer and some sunscreen, even on days the sun doesn't shine. Many French women, myself included, wear dark glasses whenever outdoors. It prevents fine lines while enhancing our mystery.

AGES FIFTY-FIVE TO SEVENTY-SEVEN . . . PLUS

With increased life expectancies, this stage, dismissed as old age just a few decades ago, is now for many one of the most vital times of life. (Better late than never.) Well-being, while not rare, is more fragile in these years, when health problems that might roll off a younger woman's back can have much more serious effects. For this reason, pampering oneself is important. You must acknowledge the positive form of "selfishness," which is not self-absorption, but a more refined and serene attentiveness to needs, comforts, and now limitations of the body. After fifty, most women have the good fortune of clearly recognizing the things they truly care about. It's a time in life when we focus on those things, improve our lives through simplification, and get real about the things to be let go. In some ways, it's when we learn to say no, not out of self-denial, but because we know better. The mind is never a stronger ally in wellness. Take it easy. This does not mean spending the rest of your days in sweats. It is the time to be not *négligée* (in the sense of negligent, rather than underwear), but soignée (elegant and groomed).

This time can be full of pleasure, but graceful aging requires some sensible renouncements. In a society obsessed with youth—always has been, but it used to be twenty-year-olds, not preteens—that's not always easy and will require all the resources of self-awareness you have cultivated. Aging can be a crisis for any woman, but those who do it well are those who end up accepting it as natural. Mourning youth is perfectly natural, too, but some, like Hamlet, mourn too long. Acceptance is rewarded with the realization that life can go on wonderfully well.

The well-tempered mind is what saves us from dwelling too much on the past (regret and loss) or the future (no longer unlimited). The same mind and breathing exercises that we use to regulate proper eating help us concentrate on the moment and living properly. These years must be taken a day at a time. Every day is a bonus. With acceptance of one's age and time remaining come gifts: a wise reluctance to waste little moments of happiness (whose preciousness the young often fritter), peace of mind that comes with tolerance, and patience with and less resentment of the world. If you do it right, time (which might seem an enemy) will seem more an illusion.

Physically, the worst offense is trying to be *une vieille qui veut faire jeune* (an older woman who decks herself out like a young thing): miniskirts, bikinis, too much makeup. They are not unheard of in France, where occasionally the well-preserved fall prey to the temptation of flaunting it. But there's nothing lovely about a seventy-year-old woman at the market in short shorts, no matter how great her legs are. Modesty is de rigueur the more impractical it becomes to conceal one's age. At that point, being natural is the best revenge. Surgery and rouge pots suggest one is not *bien dans sa peau,* which as we say is the essence of a French woman's mystique.

The French rightly acknowledge there is a particular mystique to *une femme d'un certain âge,* an expression with layers of meaning, including respect but also worldliness and hints of seduction. Our media have no trouble projecting the sexiness of Catherine Deneuve and Charlotte Rampling. Here the difference between France and America is amazing. In Europe, men naturally find women of this age group desirable, even sexy, and are often caught turning around to look at one entering a restaurant. If she is eating alone, they are more likely to flirt with her than pity her. It's inconceivable in New York, where eye contact seems to have gone the way of smoking.

If you are alert, aging seems to present you with its own commonsense instructions. But here are some adjustments to consider:

- Practice some routine physical exertion all your life, and you'll be in better shape to continue. But if you haven't, it truly is never too late to start. And the little stroll, which may have seemed a trivial improvement to your younger self, may seem more a life-affirming ritual, a reliable daily accomplishment.

- Revisit your food selection, and revise again in favor of more fruits and vegetables. Have fruit, especially berries, at least twice a day in season. Try to keep meat to once a week and fish to twice a week; eggs are fine, but no more than one a day; have lentils, green vegetables and salads, potatoes (avoid mashed and fries), brown rice, and, *bien sûr,* a glass or two of wine a day. Keep eating yogurt religiously.

- Meals and portions tend to get smaller automatically as the older body reaches satiety faster. Sometimes the problem is eating not too much but too little and suffering deficiencies. When one is having meat and fish, four to six ounces is sufficient for good nutrition, and even three is fine. Use your little scale to recalibrate your ideas of portion size. Adding the afternoon *goûter* is a good idea. A simple flan is a good source of protein and calcium. In fact, you may want to out-French the French and consider five smaller meals instead of three standard-size ones. Because their taste buds are no longer as sharp, seniors grow bored with their foods more quickly. It makes more sense to eat smaller portions than to force-feed a diet more appropriate for a younger woman, as sometimes happens.

- Be attentive to how easily you digest. Rich desserts may no longer like you as much as you like them. Reserve them for special occasions and have little portions.

- Lubricate skin morning and night. Don't forget your hands—moisturize after every wash. (Old-fashioned Vaseline Intensive Care Lotion is fine. No need for outrageously expensive creams with genetically engineered ingredients.) Another remarkably therapeutic change: Add one tablespoon of walnut oil to your daily diet. Studies have suggested benefits for mood, blood flow, and heart rhythm; and it's also an anti-inflammatory. This would have interested my relatives in Provence, who recognized this stuff as a magic potion. They used walnut and hazelnut oils frequently, but sparingly (they're expensive), on salads throughout life. Both are also wonderful new flavors if you haven't tried them.

· Water, water, water! I know I am harping, but when one has experienced eighty years of living, hydration is a life-and-death matter. When my mother reached her nineties, her doctor—not Dr. Miracle, alas, but of the same school—reminded me that at her stage, the two greatest dangers can be dehydration and sudden weight loss. *"Je n'ai pas soif"* ("I'm not thirsty") is a common refrain among the elderly, but following his instructions, she emptied one glass every three hours.

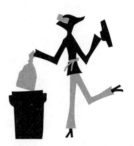

12 *bis*

Leslie, a friend from New York who loves to visit Paris, joined me for dinner recently at a luscious restaurant in the rue des Grands-Augustins, just by the Seine. As she picked at her meal, watching me eat all of mine, she told me about her lunch that afternoon. She and another American friend had been shopping till they dropped on the fashionable Faubourg St. Honoré and stopped for lunch at a trendy little bistro in the rue Matignon. Two typically done Parisian women, trimly coutured, sat at the next table. Leslie's friend said, "Watch this," confident that the two would order mesclun and Evian, having only Gauloises for the rest of lunch. Leslie was impressed to see her friend proved wrong when the ladies, nonsmokers apparently, ordered appetizers, main courses, and wine. But the Americans were floored when the French ladies tucked into an order of profiteroles for dessert while Leslie and her friend were settling their bill for the one-course lunch. "Oh well, it's genetic," her friend sniped finally.

No, it isn't. And you can be sure that those French ladies intently enjoying the pleasures of a full meal on a beautiful day were doing so entirely mindful of a compensation that would be made that evening or the next day. *C'est la vie.*

With all due respect to Watson and Crick, the capacity to enjoy food and not get fat is available to the great majority not blessed with special DNA. In fact, there are far fewer naturally tall or thin women in France than in California, Texas, or Sweden, for that matter. The real reason French women don't get fat is not genetic, but cultural, and if the French subjected themselves to the American extremes of eating and dieting, the obesity problem in France would be much worse than what has struck America. With our relatively small frames, we'd be a nation of five-by-fives rolling along the boulevards, and given my job, I would be out in front!

There is a "French Paradox" that extends far beyond the capacity to enjoy wine and cheese while preserving a healthy heart. Really, as with all paradoxes, the contradiction is only an impression that conceals a perfectly logical truth. French women don't get fat because they have not allowed new attitudes and modern theories of how the body uses food to overrule centuries of experience. They see no contradiction in eating bread and chocolate, having a bit of wine, and so on and remaining not only slender, but healthy. They do, however, understand that each of us is the keeper of her own balance, and when that balance slips, each must devise her own plan of correction, based on personal preferences. Ordinarily, the French are not ones to let a loss of balance get too far out of hand. Excess is typically a matter of a couple of days, which can be corrected in a couple of days to follow. If you plan your eating pleasures and compensations on a weekly basis, it's hard to stray too far. American women I know tend to get defeated by lapses: "Oh well, I've blown the diet, might as well go for broke." A basic failure of logic. We're all human; we all stray and return. French women do it, too. They simply understand better than others how to make amends.

Sometimes, even French women gain more weight than can be offset by a week of compensations. We too go through puberty, pregnancy, menopause—all the familiar equilibrium busters. The difference is in how we respond. The answer is never "dieting" in the American sense, but rather little alterations made steadily over time. So when we do lose the excess weight, not only does the effort seem painless, the results are much more likely to last. If my fellow Americans could adopt even a fraction of the French attitude about food and life (don't worry, you don't have to sign on to the politics, too), managing weight would cease to be a terror, an obsession, and reveal its true nature as part of the art of living.

I wouldn't be honest if I didn't confess to knowing a French woman or two who was fat all her life. We had a great family friend called Yvonne, who reveled in food and wine more than almost anyone else I have known. What excitement it was, both vicarious and actual, to share a meal with her, which I did many times before her death some years ago at the age of eighty-four. Yvonne knew she was not svelte, but her shape did not develop from a loss of control. Particularly after eighty, she simply had learned to derive so much genuine pleasure from food and drink, such a sense of vitality, that the payoff of typical compensations didn't measure up in her mind. It wasn't that she was always gaining weight; she had of her own free will set her equilibrium higher than that of most women, and she loved every day of her life. She was unusual in body, but in her spirit she could not have been more French.

My strategy with this book has also been unapologetically French. Essayistic, *bien sûr*, but incremental, too. I've tried to expose the reader bit by bit to the secrets of why French women, with rare exceptions, don't get fat. Unlike a book about diet, mine does not allow you to open to a color-coded graphic—do a, b, c, d—and get immediately to work. Really, that's part of the point. You could speed-read your way through *Madame Bovary*, picking up plot, characters, and setting, but the only way to absorb the book's insights is to surrender to the narrative, allowing that you may not see everything on the first attempt. Developing a program that will serve you a lifetime is not an instant fix. Attitude shifts take much longer, but when they take, they tend to take for good.

It would be contrary to French sensibilities to attempt to summarize or reduce a whole philosophy to a set of discrete principles. Any real design for living is more than the sum of its parts. But I'm an American, too, and being a CEO, have a particular weakness for bullets and power points. Besides, what book could call itself French if it didn't at least flirt with deconstructing itself? So with careful appreciation for the slipperiness of generalizations, the American in me feels compelled to observe that

- French women typically think about good things to eat. American women typically worry about bad things to eat.

- French women eat smaller portions of more things. American women eat larger portions of fewer things.
- French women eat more vegetables.
- French women eat a lot more fruit.
- French women love bread and would never consider a life without carbs.
- French women don't eat "fat-free," "sugar-free," or anything artificially stripped of natural flavor. They go for the real thing in moderation.
- French women love chocolate, especially the dark, slightly bitter, silky stuff with its nutty aroma.
- French women eat with all five senses, allowing less to seem like more.
- French women balance their food, drink, and movement on a week-by-week basis.
- French women do stray, but they always come back, believing there are only detours and no dead ends.
- French women don't often weigh themselves, preferring to keep track with their hands, eyes, and clothes: "zipper syndrome."
- French women eat three meals a day.
- French women don't snack all the time.
- French women never let themselves be hungry.
- French women never let themselves feel stuffed.
- French women train their taste buds, and those of their young, from an early age.
- French women honor mealtime rituals and never eat standing up or on the run. Or in front of the TV.
- French women don't watch much TV.
- French women don't have much TV to watch.

- French women eat and serve what's in season, for maximum flavor and value, and know availability does not equal quality.
- French women love to discover new flavors and are always experimenting with herbs, spices, and citrus juices to make a familiar dish seem new.
- French women eschew extreme temperatures in what they consume, and enjoy fruits and vegetables bursting with flavor at room temperature, at which they prefer their water, too.
- French women don't care for hard liquor.
- French women do enjoy wine regularly, but with meals and only a glass (or maybe two).
- French women get a kick from Champagne, as an aperitif or with food, and don't need a special occasion to open a bottle.
- French women drink water *all day long.*
- French women choose their own indulgences and compensations. They understand that little things count, both additions and subtractions, and that as an adult everyone is the keeper of her own equilibrium.
- French women enjoy going to market.
- French women plan meals in advance and think in terms of menus (a list of little dishes) even at home.
- French women think dining in is as sexy as dining out.
- French women love to entertain at home.
- French women care enormously about the presentation of food. It matters to them how you look at it.
- French women walk everywhere they can.
- French women take the stairs whenever possible.

- French women will dress to take out the garbage (you never know).
- French women are stubborn individuals and don't follow mass movements.
- French women adore fashion.
- French women know one can go far with a great haircut, a bottle of Champagne, and a divine perfume.
- French women know *l'amour fait maigrir* (love is slimming).
- French women avoid anything that demands too much effort for too little pleasure.
- French women love to sit at a café and do nothing but enjoy the moment.
- French women love to laugh.
- French women eat for pleasure.
- French women don't diet.
- French women don't get fat.

In the end, the only thing really dividing French and American women is inertia. For there is absolutely no French trick or custom that you can't make your own with a little common sense and attention to your individual needs, strengths, and weaknesses—and pleasures.

Here's your toughest challenge. Write down everything you eat this week. Don't say to yourself, "I'll remember, I don't need to write it down." Passivity won't launch you on your way. If you can take the first small step of putting pen to paper regularly and get to know what you are putting into your body, you will find yourself already en route.

Bon courage, bonne chance, and *bon appétit.*

A NOTE ABOUT THE AUTHOR

Born and raised in France, Mireille Guiliano first lived in the United States as an exchange student and came back for good early in her professional career. She is president and CEO of Clicquot, Inc., whose headquarters are in New York, and a director of Champagne Veuve Clicquot in Reims. Married to an American, Mireille lives most of the year in New York and makes frequent trips to Paris as well as across America. Among her favorite pastimes are breakfast, lunch, and dinner.

A NOTE ON THE TYPE

This book was set in a typeface called Cochin, named for Charles Nicolas Cochin the younger, an eighteenth-century French engraver. Unlike many of his contemporaries, Cochin was as much an engraver as a designer, and was deeply interested in the technique of the art. Mr. Henry Johnson first arranged for the cutting of the Cochin type in America, to be used in *Harper's Bazaar.*

Composed by North Market Street Graphics,
Lancaster, Pennsylvania
Printed and bound by R.R. Donnelley & Sons,
Harrisonburg, Virginia
Illustrated by R. Nichols
Designed by Gabriele Wilson